ANA KLIKOVAC

Bach Flower Remedies

for a Happy and Balanced Life

Foreword by Anita Moorjani

Dear Christine,

Thank you for your guidance on
my Level 1 journey! ♡
With best wishes 🌸
Ana Klikovac

B. JAIN PUBLISHERS (P) LTD.

Zagreb, 5.1.2022.   See P. 292. ♡

Ana Klikovac PhD

Bach Flower Remedies for a Happy and Balanced Life

Publisher: B. JAIN Publishers (P) LTD

Original title: Bachove kapi za sretan i uravnotežen život

Publisher of Croatian edition: Beletra, Zagreb

Year of publication: 2021

Translation from Croatian: Slavica Košća-Vrlazić

English-language editing: Lynn Brown

Cover design: Pictoris d.o.o., Zagreb, Croatia

Graphic design: Kata Ivanković Marić, Naklada Nika, Zagreb, Croatia

Cover photos © Helena Klikovac and Eva Klikovac

Published by Kuldeep Jain for
B. JAIN PUBLISHERS (P) LTD.
D-157, Sector-63, NOIDA-201307, U.P. (INDIA)
Tel.: +91-120-4933333 • *Email:* info@bjain.com
Website: **www.bjainbooks.com**
Registered office: 1921/10, Chuna Mandi, Paharganj,
New Delhi-110 055 (India)

Printed in India

ISBN: 978-81-319-2155-5

ANA KLIKOVAC PhD

Bach Flower Remedies

for a Happy and Balanced Life

Foreword by Anita Moorjani

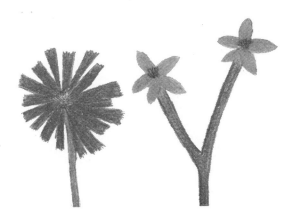

To my husband and children, who are my Sun,
and the Moon and stars

CONTENT

DISCLAIMER OF MEDICAL ADVICE

By using this book, you understand and acknowledge the terms of this disclaimer for all possible medical advice below.

The purpose of this book is not medical consultation and it does not provide medical advice.

This book contains general information on the possible application of Bach flower remedies. This information is not medical advice and should not be treated as such. The contents of this book are not intended to replace professional medical advice, diagnosis or treatment. Never disregard medical advice, discontinue treatment or delay seeking professional medical attention because of something you have read in this book.

The author and the publisher are not responsible or liable for any advice, course of treatment, diagnosis, or other information, services or products obtained by way of this book. Consult your doctor or pharmacist about the information provided in this book.

The author and the publisher assume no responsibility for the results or consequences of any attempt to use or apply any of the information contained in this book.

DISCLAIMER OF CASES AND CLIENT IMPRESSIONS

The testimonials and impressions of clients obtained by the author and used as examples in this book have been received from clients verbally or in writing. These are actual individual experiences of clients who have used the author's services, or attended her trainings, workshops and/or seminars.

Keep in mind that these are individual cases and that results will vary from person to person. The book does not claim that the results it presents are those that other individuals will achieve by using Bach flower remedies or the author's services. The statements presented herein are not necessarily examples of the results that can be expected by all those who use the described products and/or services.

The author and the publisher are not responsible for the opinions or comments expressed by the clients and used for the purposes of this book. These statements are not intended to be used as claims that these products and services may be used to diagnose, treat, cure, alleviate or prevent any physical or mental illness.

The impressions and results in the cases of clients described have not been clinically proven or evaluated by relevant institutions.

Client names and other specific customer information that might disclose identity have not been published in this book, and customer impressions have been modified to preserve client privacy and identity.

Special thanks to Stefan Ball, director of the Bach Centre, for reading this book thoroughly, word for word, and giving me his expert suggestions and comments on the text.

FOREWORD BY ANITA MOORJANI

I have been deeply touched by the contents of this book that you are holding in your hands, and even more so by my personal friendship with Ana Klikovac.

Ana came into my life through a series of events related to the late, great Dr. Wayne Dyer.

Some of you may be familiar with my story of dealing with an advanced cancer, which took me to death's door and beyond. I had a near-death experience (NDE) in 2006. I had been very sick with cancer and had tumors throughout my lymphatic system. I went into a coma and my family were called for because the doctors didn't expect me to survive very long.

But while my body was close to death, I was very much alive. I felt myself as separate from my body, and it felt like I continued to exist, as a spirit, or soul. At one point I felt myself expand so much that in fact I felt myself to be the whole universe as a state of consciousness. Among many things I felt and understood during this experience, one thing was immediately relevant to my life.

I understood that cancer in my body was a manifestation of my own energy that had turned inwards on itself. This is not to say that such a thing is true for anybody else, as we are all unique in our own ways. But I had very little self-love or self-esteem. I had lived most of my life on other people's terms. I was not living as my true authentic self.

I understood that I (and all of us) are divine expressions of consciousness, and that I had never realized this before, until now. This had caused me to always suppress my true nature. I learned that if I chose to come back into my body and to love myself, uninhibited, unreservedly, to express my authentic self from that moment onwards, then I would recover from cancer. I also understood that many diseases that we suffer from do not start at the physical level. They start from our consciousness – from our fears, stresses and our lack of belief in our own true worth.

Thankfully, I survived and lived to tell the tale of my sojourn in the other realm.

Some years after this event, Wayne Dyer discovered my story, encouraged me to write a book, and introduced me to his vast audience. I travelled the world, often sharing the stage with him.

During one of my solo tours after Wayne had passed, I was blessed to meet Ana in the audience of one of my events in the beautiful country of Croatia.

At this event, I had mentioned to my audience that I was feeling somewhat tired, due to all the travel and jet lag.

Upon hearing this, Ana sent me a beautiful gift of Bach flower remedies and homeopathic remedies that she knew would help me to feel better. On receiving this gift, I requested to meet with Ana so that she could explain to me how to use these beautiful little vials containing these 'magical elixirs'. I was excited to learn as much as I could about these remedies. And thus began my friendship with Ana.

Ana told me that she had been a huge fan of Wayne Dyer, and had read his books and followed his work – and that she had heard of me through him. We also spoke about the many synchronicities that had occurred to bring us together, and during our conversation one thing became clear. We felt that somehow, from beyond the veil, Wayne had orchestrated for us to have this time together, to get to know each other and seal our friendship.

Over the years, through my friendship with Ana, not only have I learned about the magical properties of Bach flower remedies and homeopathy, I've also learned about what a truly gifted practitioner Ana is.

You see, healing modalities like these are close to my heart, because they get to the root of the problem, and don't just treat the symptoms. They address both the physical as well as the emotional/spiritual component at the same time. After my own experience with illness and subsequent understanding of why I became ill, it became important for me that physical symptoms are treated from their root cause, instead of only managing physical symptoms through pharmaceuticals. So, over the years, as I dealt with the various ailments that befall our human bodies, Ana became my 'go to' person to ask about which remedies would best be suited for me. And each time, I would notice how intuitive she was, and how thorough, and also I marveled at how deep and detailed her understanding of this art form was. She was truly born to do this work!

Recently, when Ana told me that she was going to write a book in English on her understanding of Bach flower remedies, I was delighted, because I felt it was something I would not only be able to read myself, but could also recommend to others. And when she asked whether I would write the foreword, I was honored.

I asked her whether she was going to include her personal journey in the book, and at first she was resistant. 'Why would people be interested in my journey? They want to learn about the essences.' But I feel that you cannot truly understand Ana's work without understanding Ana's journey. You see, it took a lot for her to get to where she is today – and where she is today is truly remarkable and noteworthy. Her journey gives her work context and an immense amount of credibility. I would say she is one of the best in her field that I have had the honor to meet, and I trust her advice implicitly – and that's because I know her journey. I know she was born to do this. Over the years, she has received multiple credentials and accolades, all of which are well deserved. She has put hours of hard labor and research into her work, so for her this has been a marriage of an art form as well as a science.

In the first part of this beautiful book, you will get to know Ana as she shares the story of her life with uncommon candor. What I love about Ana is that she doesn't hold back on sharing her true self, with vulnerability. In these pages, you will get to know a woman who is both strong and sensitive, and you will also get to know a little bit about her beautiful family. She also touches on the life story of Edward Bach and the Bach Centre in the UK.

In the second part of the book, she shares her knowledge on the remedies, and she brings them to life with real-life case studies, taken from her own experience. Through these case studies, the reader can truly get a deeper understanding of the kind of intuition and depth of knowledge that is required to crack each case. Sometimes, it almost seems like Ana has to play detective to arrive at a solution and recommend the appropriate remedy – something she is really good at, because of her high intuition.

I am delighted to play a small role in helping to share Ana's work with the world. I hope you enjoy getting to know the beautifully intrinsic world of Bach flower remedies, as well as getting to know Ana through her words, as much as I did.

With love,
Anita Moorjani

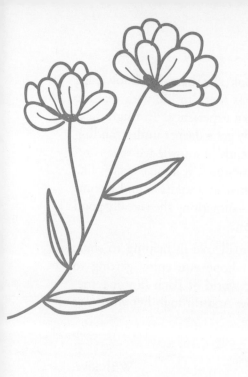

PART ONE

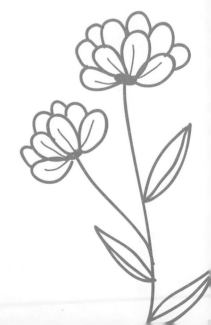

'Healing with the clean, pure, beautiful agents of Nature is surely the one method of all which appeals to most of us, and deep down in our inner self, surely there is something about it that rings true indeed: something which tells us – this is Nature's way and is right.'

Dr. Edward Bach, *The Wallingford Lectures*, 1936

LIST OF ALL 38 BACH FLOWER REMEDIES WITH LATIN NAMES AND INDICATIONS FOR APPLICATION

In this book you will be introduced to 38 Bach flower remedies.

Throughout the entire book, I will use the English names of individual flower remedies, so that readers can search for and procure them according to the names that are used universally around the world. It is not common in the literature to translate the names of flower remedies, because the bottles are usually sold under their English names in many parts of the world. Some countries, and some practitioners, like to name the flower remedies after their ordinal numbers, although this is not common practice. The ordinal numbers of the flower remedies can also be seen on the bottles.

For ease of orientation, in Table 1 you will find the names of the flower remedies in English, along with the original Latin and modern name of each plant.

List of Bach flower remedies in English and Latin, with a description of possible applications

Ordinal number	BACH FLOWER REMEDIES	APPLICATION	LATIN NAME OF PLANT, AS STATED IN DR. BACH'S WRITINGS	MODERN NAME
1	**Agrimony**	Hiding worries and problems behind a happy face	*Agrimonia Eupatoria*	
2	**Aspen**	Unknown fears	*Populus Tremula*	
3	**Beech**	Intolerance	*Fagus Sylvatica*	
4	**Centaury**	Inability to say 'no'	*Erythraea Centaurium*	*Centaurium umbellatum*
5	**Cerato**	Lack of trust in one's own decisions	*Ceratostigma Willmottiana*	*Ceratostigma willmottianum*
6	**Cherry Plum**	Fear of losing control and sanity	*Prunus Cerasifera*	
7	**Chestnut Bud**	Constant repetition of the same mistakes	*Aesculus Hippocastanum*	
8	**Chicory**	Selfish and possessive love	*Cichorium Intybus*	

9	**Clematis**	Excessive daydreaming about the future	*Clematis Vitalba*	
10	**Crab Apple**	For cleansing, self-loathing, disgust, fear of infection	*Pyrus Malus*	*Malus sylvestris*
11	**Elm**	Overburdened with responsibilities	*Ulmus Campestris*	*Ulmus procera*
12	**Gentian**	Discouragement after a setback	*Gentiana Amarella*	
13	**Gorse**	Loss of hope, despair	*Ulex Europaeus*	
14	**Heather**	Excessive self-centredness	*Calluna Vulgaris*	
15	**Holly**	Hatred, envy and jealousy	*Ilex Aquifolium*	
16	**Honeysuckle**	Excessive thinking about the past	*Lonicera Caprifolium*	
17	**Hornbeam**	Tiredness at the very thought of doing something	*Carpinus Betulus*	
18	**Impatiens**	Impatience	*Impatiens Royleii*	*Impatiens glandulifera*
19	**Larch**	Lack of self-confidence	*Larix Europaea*	*Larix decidua*
20	**Mimulus**	Everyday fears, from familiar things	*Mimulus Luteus*	*Mimulus guttatus*
21	**Mustard**	Depression that occurs for no reason	*Sinapis Arvensis*	
22	**Oak**	Overwork beyond one's endurance limits	*Quercus Pedunculata*	*Quercus robur*

23	**Olive**	Fatigue after mental or physical effort	*Olea Europaea*	
24	**Pine**	Feeling of guilt	*Pinus Sylvestris*	—
25	**Red Chestnut**	Over-concern for the welfare of loved ones	*Aesculus Carnea*	
26	**Rock Rose**	Panic and fright	*Helianthemum Vulgare*	*Helianthemum nummularium*
27	**Rock Water**	Self-imposed restrictions, rigid attitudes, self-punishment		
28	**Scleranthus**	Inability to make a decision	*Scleranthus Annuus*	
29	**Star of Bethlehem**	Shock	*Ornithogalum Umbellatum*	
30	**Sweet Chestnut**	Extreme mental anguish, feeling of having no way out	*Castanea Vulgaris*	*Castanea sativa*
31	**Vervain**	Excessive enthusiasm	*Verbena Officinalis*	
32	**Vine**	Domination over others and inflexibility	*Vitis Vinifera*	
33	**Walnut**	Protection from unwanted influences of others and help with adjustment in periods of change	*Juglans Regia*	
34	**Water Violet**	Self-built barrier between us and others, leading to loneliness	*Hottonia Palustris*	

35	**White Chestnut**	Unwanted thoughts that cause rumi-nation and mental torture	*Aesculus Hippocastanum*	
36	**Wild Oat**	Uncertainty when choosing a life direction	*Bromus Asper*	*Bromus ramosus*
37	**Wild Rose**	Defeatism, resignation to destiny, listlessness	*Rosa Canina*	
38	**Willow**	Self-pity, rancour, resentment	*Salix Vitellina*	

Note: In this table, and in Table 2 later in the book, I have retained Dr. Bach's usage, which is to present plants' Latin names with an initial capital on the second word as well as the first. In the rest of the book, however, I have adopted the current accepted convention, which is for the second word in each term to be presented wholly in lower-case letters.

It is important to note the following in the list of flower remedies:

- The Bach flower remedies system consists of 37 flower essences plus spring water as a special essence.

- The Chestnut Bud and White Chestnut flower remedies are prepared from the same wild chestnut tree (lat. *Aesculus hippocastanum*), but the essence itself is made at different stages of flowering. The flower essence for the Chestnut Bud remedy is prepared from a flower bud, and the White Chestnut flower essence from a wild chestnut flower.

INTRODUCTION AND MY STORY

This is no ordinary manual on Bach flower remedies. My idea was to write a book that would bring flower remedies to life for the reader, by showing how much they mean to me and how much they have changed my life. Without my story, readers would not be able to get an idea of the extent to which I felt it was my mission to write this book. It would not be clear how much these flower remedies speak themselves through me. And that is why I have included my story here as well. I was encouraged to do so by my dear friend Anita Moorjani, a famous author about whom I write in more detail later in this introduction. She told me: 'People need to hear your story!' And where better to incorporate my story than into a book about Bach flower remedies – a method that completely transformed and brightened my life.

This book is a story of the unique and miraculous 38 flower remedies that change lives and destinies. And that is why I wish to first tell you what Bach flower remedies mean to me personally. As a true Vervain type, I am penning my story to convince you of the power and beauty of this method, hoping to convert you, to bring well-being and joy into your life so that you yourself would embark on the path of using Bach flower remedies. All the better if I convince some of you to take the road of education about Bach flower remedies and become Bach practitioners or teachers yourselves! With this story, I take the opportunity to convince you of the miraculousness of these flower remedies. And it will be a great honour to hear one day how much this book has transformed you, how much it has helped you, how much you have found your happiness and peace with its help. That is why I am telling this story and that is why I am writing this book!

Do not be surprised that in this introductory part I often mention homeopathy as part of my journey and what I do. Let us remember that Dr. Bach was also a homeopath and that his idea of a simple healing system emanated precisely from his experiences with homeopathy. In his works, and in particular in *Ye Suffer from Yourselves*, he wrote about homeopathy. He repeatedly mentioned Dr. Samuel Hahnemann, the founder of homeopathy. Even Dr. Bach's collaborator, Nora Weeks, in her biography of Dr. Bach, chose Dr. Hahnemann's quote as an introductory quote for the book. Dr. Bach also practised homeopathy in one part of his life. Today, I practise it too. It is complementary to Bach flower remedies, so it is a part of this story of mine that cannot be omitted. But, except for my introduction, the rest of the book is dedicated exclusively to Bach flower remedies.

Let us start, then. This is my story ...

WHO AM I TODAY?

Today I am a registered Bach flower practitioner and teacher, licensed by The Bach Centre in England. I work according to the principles and the Code of Ethics of Dr. Edward Bach, and I am the first Croatian teacher for Bach flower remedies. I completed all my training on Bach flower remedies directly at The Bach Centre.

I am a homeopath and I have my own homeopathy centre, 'Annah', in Zagreb, Croatia, where I offer counselling and education on Bach flower remedies, homeopathy and other related methods.

I am a lecturer and a representative of the homeopathic academy 'The Other Song', in India. I give lectures in person at the academy in Mumbai or via its online programmes. In cooperation with the same academy, for the first time in Europe we are organising training on homeopathy in Zagreb within my homeopathic centre, where I give half of all the lectures, while the other half are taught by Indian lecturers. I specialise in lectures in the field of the Organon (the basic work of homeopathy), the *Materia Medica* of homeopathic remedies and the Sensation Method in homeopathy. I give lectures in Croatian or English, depending on whether I have a domestic or international group of students. I am currently finishing two books on homeopathy in English.

I am a collaborator of Dr. Rajan Sankaran, a distinguished Indian homeopath with international reach, and a visionary whose methods and works have enriched and expanded homeopathic practice. I am the owner of ASHUH, whose mission is to promote homeopathy and related methods, and to organise international lectures, seminars and congresses in collaboration with Dr. Sankaran. Thus, despite the global crisis caused by the Covid-19 virus, in November 2020 I organised an online seminar for Synergy Homeopathic, originally planned for presentation in Zagreb, which brought together world-renowned homeopaths to share their best experiences from practice.

I am a consultant for Schuessler salts and facial analysis, and was the first in Croatia to offer certified training for counsellors in facial analysis, which has so far been attended by many participants from Croatia, Slovenia, Bosnia and Herzegovina, Serbia, Montenegro, Germany, Austria, India, the United States of America and numerous other countries, including doctors, pharmacists, pharmaceutical technicians, veterinarians and medical staff.

I was the first in Croatia to complete practitioner training for Australian Bush Flower Essences and the Buteyko breathing method, and subsequently made these methods available to those who would benefit from their help.

To achieve all this, I flew across half the world, saving neither money nor time, knowing that I was investing in my own future, as well as that of my family, my children, their children, the well-being of all those who would learn these methods from me, in Croatia and elsewhere.

I studied Bach flower remedies in England, where I have travelled five times to date, each time taking the opportunity to visit the local cemetery where Dr. Edward Bach is buried, to thank him over and over again for his life-changing method. The energy in The Bach Centre is special. The atmosphere is inexpressible – you sit on a bench in the middle of the garden, surrounded by Bach flowers, of which Chicory, Agrimony and Honeysuckle notably stand out, while Mimulus rises by the water in front of you; you hear only the sound of the breeze, beautiful birds fly in the sky – the red kite,[1] whose flight is magnificent and which I could watch for hours. And the realisation that Dr. Bach lived in that house, that everything was established there, that everything started from there, gives you the feeling that you are finally at home. Peace, quiet, repose, flowers and learning – this is what awaits you at The Bach Centre.

I learned the Buteyko method in Ireland, travelling across the country during my clinical practice in Dublin, Cork and Galway.

I studied homeopathy for two years in Zagreb, within the school for French and classical homeopathy. After completing my education, I advanced my skills all over the world, with the world's leading homeopaths. Thus, on several occasions, I have stayed at India's The Other Song academy in Mumbai, where I performed clinical practice and perfected my education in the field of the Sensation Method and the 8-Box Method. Nowadays, I am a faculty member at that Indian academy, as well as a contractual representative for the Republic of Croatia, but also for the wider region.

I studied almost all approaches and methods in homeopathy, in order to acquire the most extensive knowledge possible of all available homeopathic approaches – the French, the clinical and classical method, and the modern approaches to homeopathy.

I studied several different programmes at the academy for classical homeopathy in Greece, where I also studied the Organon. In the Netherlands I learned from Jan Scholten his method of working with plant remedies in homeopathy. Also in the Netherlands, I completed my training in the detox method of homeopathy and CEASE therapy for the ap-

---

[1]   Milvus milvus.

plication of homeopathy in autism cases, and was included in the Dutch registers of counsellors in these methods.

I am proud to have had the honour of meeting the late Dr. Prasanta Banerji, and his son Dr. Pratip Banerji, the founders of the Dr. Prasanta Banerji Homeopathic Research Foundation in Calcutta, India, and hearing and learning directly from them about the Banerji Protocols in homeopathy.

THE SEARCH FOR KNOWLEDGE IN THE US AND GERMANY

I was especially interested in the history and development of homeopathy, and for years I independently studied the work of the founder of homeopathy, Dr. Samuel Hahnemann, and that of other great historical figures of homeopathy. I devoted most of my time to studying the work of the German physician Dr. Constantine Hering, who expanded homeopathy teachings to the United States in the early 19th century, where he emigrated in 1833 from Germany, his homeland.

According to Dr. Hahnemann, Dr. Hering was his favourite, due to his numerous contributions to homeopathy, including the establishment of the first homeopathic college in Allentown and Philadelphia in the United States. Personally, in my practice, I am guided by the most comprehensive *materia medica* in homeopathy – Hering's *The Guiding Symptoms of Our Materia Medica*, which is written in ten volumes.

I was so very much interested in the history of homeopathy because I knew that I would discover in historical writings the foundations of this method and develop the best understanding of the working methods of the greatest homeopaths in history. Similarly, I felt I had to visit the locations where they worked and lived at the time, so I could additionally feel that energy and adopt as much knowledge as possible from these great masters.

I visited Dr. Samuel Hahnemann's house in Koethen, Germany, where I had the opportunity to see his study, the set of homeopathic remedies exhibited on his desk, and the garden where he liked to sit, in which he wrote his work *The Chronic Diseases* and where his fellow homeopaths would gather. I walked through Koethen and visited the monuments and landmarks erected in memory of Dr. Hahnemann, and saw numerous of his quotations written on the facades of houses in this charming little German town.

During my visit to Dr. Hahnemann's last resting place in Paris, I bowed to him and thanked him for his greatness and contributions, due to which today we can rapidly, gently and permanently eliminate the difficulties that afflict us.

I also travelled to Philadelphia, USA, and visited the locations where Dr. Constantine Hering lived and worked. It was an unforgettable experience to stand in the street where his house and office once stood, and where a memorial plaque has been put up in his honour, as well as in front of the building of his homeopathic college, which is also marked with a memorial plaque. Walking the same streets Dr. Hering had walked in the 19th century – the street where the first homeopathic pharmacy was opened at his initiative, the street along which he passed when he came to give lectures at the homeopathic college – and visiting major city landmarks, such as that where the Liberty Bell is exhibited, the symbol of American independence since 1752, I could feel the spirit of the time in which Dr. Constantine Hering spent his entire working life, there in the 19th century, with his family, associates and followers.

During my visit to the USA, I also travelled to Washington, DC, where one of the largest monuments to Dr. Samuel Hahnemann is located. Right under his statue, the basic homeopathic principle is carved: '*Similia Similibus Curentur*', 'Like cures like'. I felt proud that a monument to the founder of homeopathy has been erected in the capital of the United States, in the city where the White House is located.

All those experiences made me what I am today. My fundamental mission was initially to make these methods available in my homeland, Croatia, where some of these teachings were inaccessible or under-represented, and later I felt the need to pass on everything I learned to all those who wanted to learn these noble and useful methods. And that is why my mission is to lecture, to write books, to teach, mentor, talk, talk and talk about these methods.

And that is why my books are also written in English, and why I translated Dr. Bach's works from English into the Croatian language, hoping to reach as many people as possible in my mission to spread these methods.

But, before all this, I laid the foundations of my success in homeopathy by doing something completely different. And so, to continue, I will testify to who I was before, what I did before, and how I set out to learn and implement the methods that are imprinted into me today.

MY CAREER BEFORE THE TURNING POINT

I received my doctorate in 2011 at the Faculty of Economics, University of Zagreb, for my thesis titled 'The role of auditing in fraud prevention as a prerequisite of the stability of capital markets'. I received my master's degree at the same faculty in 2006, for my thesis titled 'An impact of the harmonisation of financial reporting in the European Union on financial reporting in the Republic of Croatia'. For my doctoral and master's theses, I received awards from the Croatian Association of Accountants and Financial Professionals.

In the period from 2006 to 2017 I taught courses in the field of accounting and auditing at a higher education institution, and I was head of graduate study for Accounting, Auditing and Taxes. I am a certified internal auditor, a specialist in the field of economics.

I am the author of the book *Financial Reporting in the European Union*, and of numerous papers in the field of accounting and auditing. I am co-author of a chapter in the book *Management, Governance and Entrepreneurship*, titled 'Challenges and perspectives in fraud prevention and detection for management'.

During my teaching career, I held lectures for both certified external auditors and internal auditors in banks and companies in Croatia, Serbia, and Bosnia and Herzegovina, and published a number of scientific and professional articles within the country and abroad. I was also giving lectures at professional and scientific conferences and was building my academic career.

For the purposes of the doctorate, considering that my topic was detecting fraud in auditing, I studied forensic auditing, methods of conducting investigations and interviews with fraud perpetrators, which included knowledge of body language, non-verbal and verbal communication, detection of signs of lies in communication, but also in great part knowledge of the psychology of the perpetrator of the fraud.

What is it that drives a person to commit fraud, lie and steal? I was extremely interested in this, so I went deeper and deeper into the study of personality types and psychology. Simultaneously, I studied NLP modules, communication skills in both the business and the private sector, and developed a growing interest in recognising types of people. I read books in the areas of psychology, personal development and self-help. Considering that at the time I was already to a considerable extent using my knowledge of Bach flower remedies, which also speak of personality types, I began to realise that all my teachings overlapped and complemented one another. Psychological profiles of persons can also be recognised in homeopathy, and Schuessler salts also have their basis in understanding the type of person and their reaction to stress.

I realised that all of the above have a common denominator – human behaviour, human problems, stress and reactions to stress.

I realised that all my life some higher power had led me step by step to the moment when I would one day leave economy and devote myself to counselling in the field of homeopathy, Bach flower remedies and all other methods. It was all intertwined, and created one knowledge network and database that serves me today when I work with clients who use these wonderful natural healing methods.

My former profession – economics, accounting and auditing – serves me well today in running my own companies. During Dr. Rajan Sankaran's first visit to Zagreb, in 2019, when I organised his seminar, he told me that my great strength lies in my knowledge of economics and running a business, because it is sometimes the missing link in the work of homeopaths, the consequence being that their consultation practice sometimes ends in business losses, with a negative balance, or they close their practices and give up further work with clients. Then he told me to include business counselling for homeopaths in my education programmes, training on how to run businesses and profitable homeopathic practice. I then received his invitation to teach homeopaths in India the skills of running a successful homeopathic counselling business. Thus, homeopaths I personally mentor in my courses also learn these business and communication skills from me.

Yes, my whole development path makes a lot of sense. I would not change a single step in my life. Each brought me to where I am today. And God's hand continues to lead me. And I am grateful for that!

MY PROFESSIONAL AND PERSONAL TURNING POINT

When I first decided to try Bach flower remedies, I wasn't aware how strong they were. And I didn't know that it was going to be a crucial moment that would determine the rest of my life and that that moment would transform me for ever. I did not know that.

I was 29 at the time and was on maternity leave with my second daughter, Eva. My eldest daughter, Helena, was only two years old. But, instead of enjoying my time and walking in the park with my children, I carried the burden of professional responsibility. The deadline for completing my master's degree was approaching and I was writing my master's thesis. I would usually spend the days with the children and when they fell asleep I would work on my thesis until three or four o'clock in the morning. Sometimes I would write even when they were awake. Helena used to stand in a chair right behind me, combing and doing my hair, and Eva was crawling under my desk. My husband would often take care of them entirely so I could write in peace. My father-in-law, Branko Klikovac, also took part in caring for the children almost every day. My brain was working at a hundred an hour and was overloaded. And when I did go to bed, I could not stop thinking. I would continue to write my paper in my head, or wonder if I would make it at all.

Then my friend Vesna, who knew what state I was in and what I was going through, brought me a newspaper article providing short descriptions and a list of all 38 Bach flower remedies. I will never forget that moment. I was reading the list, going one remedy at a time, and then came across the White Chestnut remedy. Wow! That was exactly what I needed! It said, 'Flower remedy for unwanted thoughts that cause mental torture and anguish to the person day and night.' I was astounded that there was a plant in this world that treated exactly the condition I was in at the time.

My first reaction was thrill and I immediately sat down at the computer to look for more information. I managed to find a lady who was probably the only one working with Bach flower remedies at the time, even though she was not a Bach practitioner, and I booked an appointment. That same day, I also ordered all available books from the Internet, in English, about Bach flower remedies.

I went to pick up the bottles of Bach flower remedies with Eva in my arms, while Helena was in kindergarten. As a real Agrimony person, being the type at the time, I wasn't ready to tell anything to that lady about myself and my problems. I gave her a piece of paper with a list of remedies for all my family members and the ingredients for each of us. Today, I remember only that my bottle contained the remedies Agrimony (my type at the time) and White Chestnut (the state of mind that bothered me at the time). I chose my own flower remedies then and that is exactly the point of Dr. Bach's system – to choose your own remedies, to get to know yourself and your loved ones better, and to find help for your own problems. Let this book serve as a guide for anyone who wants to choose their own remedies and learn more about this self-help method.

So, my first bottle contained White Chestnut flower remedy. I remember it as if it were yesterday, that feeling, when those disturbing thoughts disappeared as if taken away by hand. It was as if I had some invisible shield in my head that protected me from negative thoughts and gave me a clearer focus. I was able to fall asleep without any problems the first day after taking the flower remedies. So, the flower remedies were a miracle!

The next morning I felt some urge inside, some desire, to read and learn everything that exists in this world about these magic flower remedies. That day, I don't even know where and how, overwhelmed with enthusiasm, I recited:

- One day I will be a Bach practitioner!
- One day I will translate all of Dr. Bach's works into Croatian!
- And one day I will write my own book about Bach flower remedies!

I became a Bach practitioner almost ten years later, in 2014. That same year, I translated all of Dr. Bach's works and donated the translations to The Bach Centre, as a sort of expression of personal gratitude to Dr. Bach; and so that anyone who wants to read about Bach flower remedies can do so for free and in Croatian. At the moment, you are holding in your hands the book I wrote about Bach flower remedies.

And I actually achieved more than I had planned at the time – I also became a licensed teacher for Bach flower remedies.

But my story isn't only about that … The real transformation happened in the period between this today and my first tasting of the flower remedies.

I completed my master's degree and received an award for that work. I changed jobs and was employed at a higher education institution where I taught accounting and auditing. My career as faculty member started and the next step was to get a doctoral degree, which was dictated by the nature of my job.

CLIENT TRUST

In the meantime, I had already started using Bach flower remedies extensively, for myself, my family, friends and acquaintances, but still as a self-taught practitioner. I worked as a professor, I had a family, and I was pretty happy and content with my life.

But then the deadline by which I was supposed to receive my doctorate was approaching. I found myself in the same situation again – I was on maternity leave with my third child, my son Ante, and I was writing my doctoral thesis. This time, in addition to Bach flower remedies, I harnessed the power of homeopathy and several other alternative methods in order to withstand the weight of stress and pressure of that period. It was one of the most difficult periods of my life, when I was trying to reconcile my role as wife and mother and finish writing my dissertation. There were days when I needed Cherry Plum because sometimes I felt like throwing the computer and all the books out of the window. I would also take Gorse when I was going through days when I would rather give up writing.

However, I did finish the dissertation. Once again with exceptional achievements and praise, and an award for the work. My husband, children, my friends and family, all my loved ones, listened to the public defence of my doctoral thesis and celebrated with me at the promotion ceremony.

I have told my daughters many times since then, it is a great distress and sacrifice when a woman, who is primarily a wife and mother, needs to get a doctorate. I would not wish anyone that torment, that stress and that abnegation. And yet I am proud of my doctorate, and my motto since then has been 'endure, endure, endure'.

But I endured much more than the above.

Although the Agrimony in me would like me to keep my story written only superficially, to halt at the difficulties of the master's and doctoral dissertations, my husband encouraged me to make this an 'open book', to make it something that would help everyone who reads it and needs it. An authentic and real story. Believe me, it took me a total of four working versions of this introductory story to be able to put on paper the most painful part. What I wish I didn't need to write and that I had not had to go through. But I had. Today some of you may be going through something similar. And that is why things should be called by their proper names. And that is why I am going to include that part of the story here. Not necessarily in chronological order and not necessarily by degree of severity.

In one period of my life, I suffered from panic attacks, feared food allergies and almost ended up with anorexia because of it. Panic attacks are something terrible because you literally think you are going to die. And then the doctor tells you there is nothing wrong with you and that you are just panicking. So you start to think that you are actually going crazy. Classical medicine has no cure for that, but I deeply believed that it must be there somewhere in the world. As a true Vervain type, I searched and searched – and I found it! A recommendation of a kind doctor who was open to alternative medicine led me to the door of an alternative therapist, where I subsequently regained my balance with a combination of osteopathy and an energy method. The hours and hours and numerous days of work that I invested then in my personal development, along with countless books, prepared me for my future role as a homeopath and Bach flower remedies practitioner. This experience showed me the true strength of alternative medicine and the shortcomings of the system of classical medicine. Also, through that period, I filtered out the methods that worked best for me personally and found my own unique alternative path.

Today, I like to joke and say that with this experience I became a 'specialist' in providing help with panic attacks, and for a while, after opening my own homeopathy centre, I had hordes of people who came to me for help specifically with panic-related problems. Because, unlike the doctors, I understood them, and it was easier for them to tell their story without anyone looking at them in amazement and without telling them, 'It's nothing!'

DIVORCE HAS MADE US STRONGER

I also went through turbulent stages in my marriage. My husband Saša is my high-school sweetheart and my soulmate. I was always telling him that I ordered him 'tailor-made' and that he was born designed according to my wishes. Since he is ten months younger than me, my 'imaginary' story is that immediately after birth I wished for him to be born – my other half, my only love. And the story about how the two of us enrolled in the same school and the same class is just as unusual and involves some sort of divine intervention. The two of us meeting and falling in love when I was 15 and he was 14 years old – and having stayed together all these years to this day is nothing short of real fate. Despite that great love, we went through a phase where he felt neglected, and I on the other hand felt he did not care any more. Our mutual outstanding debts, which had accumulated over the years, became due one day, and we went through a divorce, despite the fact that neither of us really wanted it. Needless to say, I survived that period thanks to Bach flower remedies, which made that painful time easier, both for me and my children. Eventually, my then ex-husband also turned to Bach flower remedies, and also found his peace and balance. Our love was ultimately stronger than anything; the remedies worked for both of us, and after a year we remarried – in the presence of our three beautiful children. Divorce did not separate us; it only strengthened and connected us even more. When you go through a divorce like that, you realise how many people are actually throwing their days to the wind, how much they do not appreciate each other, and how much they take what they have for granted. The fact that we were separated for a while taught us gratitude, and that we should work every day on the quality of our relationship and to protect each other. He is the only one who knows my dreams, who sees my aptitude; he is my lodestar and my inspiration. In return, I try to give him the same and more every day.

I shared with Saša back in high school my dreams of a big family. Being a mum and having a lot of kids has always been my great wish. Although I do not remember it, even as a little girl I used to say that I would have a lot of children. This story was reported to me several times by my wonderful Štefica, a neighbour who looked after me when I was little and with whom I spent some of the happiest moments of my childhood. Even today I remember running after school to Štefica's place, where I was always greeted with warmth, tenderness and complete devotion to me and my juvenile concerns. She never found it hard to indulge my whims and cook a meal for me at midnight, if I happened to yearn for something. I still love and appreciate Štefica indescribably. She simply knows my heart and is always there for me, unconditionally and sincerely. Many times I recognise that it was she who instilled in me some of my deepest life and spiritual values, which taught me to be a better person and to be there for others.

HELPING YOUNG COUPLES

Pregnancy has often been my natural state. Being a mum is my biggest life achievement. Our children – Helena, Eva and Ante – are a real gift from God. That is right – God's gift. Because I realised, in a painful way, that we humans cannot always influence whether a child is born or not. It is all God's plan.

I was pregnant five times. Although all my pregnancies were wanted and planned, I gave birth to three children and three I lost. During my fourth pregnancy, I lost the twins I was carrying, in the 12th week of my pregnancy. Their hearts stopped beating. The fifth pregnancy was even worse: I went through the traumatic termination of pregnancy at 14 weeks, with a baby who reportedly had Edwards syndrome. I knew then that if I could survive the emotional pain of that event, and continue with my life, that I could endure anything. And those two experiences changed me profoundly. My children learned from this that in life you should always get up when you fall, no matter how painful it is, and that there is no giving up. I never gave up, obviously, the Gorse flower remedy did the thing, so I can say today that I did my best to try again in hopes of having more children, but God's plan for me was something else. I have a mission: to help others. And so, with exceptional joy, I try, through homeopathy and Bach flower remedies, to help those who struggle to bring a baby into the world. I believe you will notice that the topics of pregnancy and childbirth run through this book in several places. May this book and Bach flower remedies help every woman, every pregnant woman, every couple who wholeheartedly want a child.

My life would certainly have been easier had I not gone through these experiences, but I still cannot say that I wish I hadn't gone through them. Looking back, each experience had its purpose. After going through all those experiences, I was no longer the same. Because of that, I discovered another side of life and the world – I discovered the power of nature, the power of alternative methods, the power of Bach flower remedies, the power of homeopathy, but also my personal strength. And that changed my life's direction, led me to an entirely new one, which is to help all those people who are having a hard time, who are going through difficult periods in life, find the same as me – their salvation, their peace and their balance. I found my way.

It was Wild Oat flower remedy that illuminated my path and showed me what I already felt inside: my path was Bach flower remedies, homeopathy and related natural methods.

After I received my doctorate, I enrolled in all the formal training courses and completed Bach Levels 1, 2 and 3 education and teaching programmes at The Bach Centre. I completed my education in homeopathy and travelled half the world in search of knowledge. I opened my own centre for homeopathy and health support. I completely abandoned my career as an accounting and auditing professor, to do what is my true calling, my life mission, my purpose, my love: Bach flower remedies, homeopathy and related natural methods.

I should mention here that few around me understood my decision to take this new and unknown path. They tried to discourage and scare me, telling me I was crazy to take a risk and leave a 'real job' to mix some remedies. Leaving a secure job and a secure salary, for an entrepreneurial venture that is abstract and uncertain was, to most people around me, insane. They wondered what was it that I was actually going to do. But I did not allow myself to be intimidated. I believed in the purpose given to me, in the calling I recognised, in the talent I discovered in myself. My husband knew it was the 'real me' and he believed in me. To my children, my job in economics was abstract, and the world of homeopathy and Bach flower remedies, in which they grew up, was completely understandable and logical. And their support subsequently became my fuel. I started my own business and began to help others. Because of that sudden turnaround in my career, many beautiful things happened to the people around me. Some children were born although previously there were obstacles. Borna and Luka are two boys who needed a miracle – and their mothers found that miracle in Bach flower remedies. If there had been only those two cases from my practice to be taken into consideration, it was worth starting to do this!

Today I teach these methods and spread the knowledge I have gained, and that is my path – the path I took when I tried my first bottle of Bach flower remedies.

I didn't know that with these flower remedies I would go through a personal and business transformation. I didn't know which way these flower remedies would take me. All I know is that this is me now, that this is my path, that I am much stronger and more powerful, and that I am doing what I love.

WHY I WROTE THIS BOOK

As I mentioned earlier, my mission is to teach and spread the natural methods I am using today. Giving lectures and writing books are skills I acquired during my previous career. Or I got them as talents by birth. Anyway, to me teaching and writing is something completely natural and I do it with ease. I never get tired when I give lectures or when I write texts.

But I am aware that there are time, location and financial constraints that prevent all those people I need to teach from coming to me. So I concluded that I would more easily reach all those who want to learn and read about these topics if I wrote a book. And that's why I wrote this book in both Croatian and English – to make it available to anyone who needs to read it.

Numerous examples from my rich practice with clients are presented throughout the book, as well as some of my personal experiences, and I have also woven into it examples of my friends and people dear to me. I have described some of the remedies in great detail through my personal experiences. These are the flower remedies that touched me deeply, changed me and gave me some wonderful insights. We all have our favourite flower remedies, and so do I. Such flower remedies are described and coloured with tones of beauty and gratitude for the lessons they have taught me. But in my seminars I always say, you will get to know the flower remedies best only when you try them personally. Not when you read about them. Not when you recommend them to others. Not when you study them in detail. No! You need to feel the flower remedies. You need to feel the difference in the condition before using them and what you experienced, what you became or how you changed after taking them. Yes, I tried them all! All 38! Each remedy in its own time and when I needed it. And that is why I'm writing this book. To revive these flower remedies for you too, and to convey to you their beauty and wisdom.

There are no words to describe how healing this system is when you give in to the remedies. Some people fail to find themselves in it. Some say that the remedies do not help them. Some say that they make their condition worse (which is impossible, because the flower remedies work only for your well-being and in no other way). It is all resistance and non-acceptance of the change that these flower remedies bring. And it is all just fine. If now is not the time to use them, they will find you again sometime in the future when you are ready for them. Or they are there just to take you to some other method or therapy that is more convenient for you. They are there to help you if you let them and if you want to. They are there and waiting patiently if you don't want them now. But their healing power is unquestionable and indisputable.

I believe that by reading this book, you will, somewhere, find help and a solution for yourself. This is a system that is simple and unobtrusive, and yet it is there to turn your life around for the better, to save you, to get you back into balance and to help you find yourself.

Enjoy this book!

I have tried to write a book with which I would remove all your doubts regarding choosing remedies, and which would provide many examples and comparisons of similar remedies. At the same time, this book aims to help those who will embark on the path of Bach practitioners and teachers, or are already working with clients.

This was my story for you, and now you, with the help of this book and Bach flower remedies, can create your own story.

I wish you the best of luck on your journey with Bach flower remedies!

Ana Klikovac
Zagreb, 1 January 2021

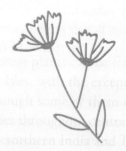

SEVEN GROUPS OF BACH FLOWER REMEDIES

In order to facilitate navigation through the Bach flower remedies system, Dr. Bach classified 38 remedies into seven groups, which apply to the following conditions and problems:

1. **For loneliness**
2. **For fear**
3. **For despondency or despair**
4. **For insufficient interest in present circumstances**
5. **For over-care for welfare of others**
6. **For those over-sensitive to influences and ideas**
7. **For uncertainty**

It is important to know, however, that knowledge of the groups is not necessary in order to choose the remedies you need.

When selecting the remedies, we can put together a maximum of seven different flower remedies in one bottle, i.e. any seven remedies we need at that moment.

In exceptional situations, an eighth remedy can be added, if necessary and if deemed that without it the person would not make progress. Dr. Bach prepared a bottle with nine remedies in just two cases during his extensive practice. So, don't use this option unless it is really needed. Because, you don't want to give your mind more assignments than the ones it is ready to process at this moment.

All remedies can be combined, even those that have a seemingly opposite effect. There is no obligation to select one from each group. There is no rule prohibiting you from using more than one flower remedy from one group. You can select any seven flower remedies from the list to prepare your personal combination. It is important to choose the flower remedies that you need <u>now</u>, for the problem that is currently bothering you.

To reiterate, groups of flower remedies exist only for ease of reference within the system, so if you find it difficult at first to remember which flower remedies belong to which group, do not be discouraged. You will learn it at some point, if you need to. Until then, it is important that you have a good understanding of the purpose of each flower remedy in order to find precisely the ones you need most. Read about them in this book, study them one by one, and in time you will master them very well. That is why I have provided a lot of examples and comparisons – to clarify how to distinguish similar flower remedies, to facilitate your screening process so you can better learn the specifics of each remedy.

I am starting with clarification of why certain flower remedies are classified into a particular group, also providing a brief description to make it easier to distinguish the flower remedies, just so you can see immediately at the beginning of the book what are the possibilities of the remedies and what you can use them for.

You can find a more detailed description of each individual remedy in the second part of the book, where I describe each flower remedy separately under an individual title.

Why are certain flower remedies classified into a particular group?

FOR LONELINESS

Heather – those who cannot stand loneliness and cannot stand being alone; they are often alone because people avoid them, because of their habit of talking too much about themselves and their problems

Impatiens – they are alone because they are not synchronised with the pace of other people; they like to do everything fast, are not a team player and prefer to do everything by themselves and at their own pace; other people's slowness angers them, as does waiting in line, and in these situations they tend to explode with anger, to quarrel and swear

Water Violet – they love being alone and choose to be alone, but this makes them lonely in the long run; they are aware of their positive qualities, so others sometimes see them as arrogant and conceited

FOR FEAR

Aspen – an undefined fear of unknown cause

Cherry Plum – fear of losing sanity, fear of madness and loss of control

Mimulus – a defined fear of known origin

Red Chestnut – fear for others, for the welfare of the people close to us

Rock Rose – panic fear with physical manifestations, such as heart palpitations, trembling hands, etc.

FOR DESPONDENCY OR DESPAIR

Crab Apple – feeling dissatisfied with their physical appearance

Elm – feeling overwhelmed because they are not able to perform all their tasks, due to the overwhelming amount of responsibility they have taken on, although they know that they are otherwise able to perform all tasks

Larch – feeling discouraged because they have no self-confidence, and do not trust their knowledge and ability to perform a task

Oak – a very responsible person who has a lot of obligations to fulfil and does not have time to rest

Pine – feeling guilt and remorse for something they have done, or taking the blame of others on to themselves

Star of Bethlehem – a person has experienced a stressful and shocking situation

Sweet Chestnut – feeling desperate because they fail to remove the suffering and pain they feel, and the condition becomes unbearable and intolerable

Willow – a person is resentful because of an unfortunate or unjust event that has befallen them

FOR INSUFFICIENT INTEREST IN PRESENT CIRCUMSTANCES

Chestnut Bud – they keep repeating the same mistakes from the past

Clematis – they are not present in the now because in their thoughts they are in the clouds and in the world of imagination, and they expect that they would be better off and happier in the future or somewhere else, or with another person

Honeysuckle – they are not present in the now because they live spiritually in the past, in times more pleasant than now

Mustard – although they have no reason for depression and bad mood, they are not happy and satisfied in the present moment and feel as if a black cloud is hovering over them

Olive – due to fatigue, they are not present in the now, as they are run-down or exhausted after a disease or after making an effort of some kind.

White Chestnut – they are not present in the now because their mind is following some parallel flow of thoughts, because they are worried, because they are going over and over some old traumas and injuries, and they cannot get rid of those thoughts

Wild Rose – they are not aware that they are just vegetating in the present moment, without enjoying life and without doing things that would make their present moment more beautiful and fulfilling

Beech – they think that they do everything best and, for the benefit of the other person, they draw that person's attention to all their flaws and the things they are doing wrong

Chicory – they want to have their loved ones with them possessively, because they think they are best off with them

Rock Water – they think that they do everything best and believe that, with a strict regime and lifestyle, they will inspire others to follow their example, so they would also have a good life

Vervain – activists, they think that their role is to save the world, the planet, other people, animals, and convince others that they should, for their own benefit, side with them, with the way they act and think

Vine – they believe that they know what is best for others, and order them how to behave, what to do and how to live

How do certain types of flower remedies express their concern for others?

Beech – <u>by criticising</u> others they want to get them on the right track

Chicory – <u>manipulates</u> others so they will act as they want and in line with what they think should be done

Rock Water – <u>tacitly, they want to show others, through their personal example</u>, how to live and work properly, hoping that others will follow their example

Vervain – <u>by convincing and persuading</u> others, they convey their beliefs and attitudes about what they are doing, because they believe that this is the best way for others as well

Vine – <u>by giving orders</u> to others they want to help them do the right thing

FOR THOSE OVER-SENSITIVE TO INFLUENCES AND IDEAS

Agrimony – they do not talk about their problems, but hide them behind a smile; they love being in fun company as this is their way to forget about their problems, and may be prone to abuse of alcohol and other vices

Centaury – they are easily manipulated by others, unable to fight for themselves, yield when asked to do something, and even though they know they should refuse, are not able to say 'no'

Holly – vindictive people, who very easily become jealous and suspicious

Walnut – although they make a decision, they are sometimes diverted from their path, so they don't stick to their decisions and commitments

FOR UNCERTAINTY

Cerato – insecure about their decisions, do not trust their own intuition, so ask others for advice

Gentian – after a setback, they are discouraged and think they will fail, having previously failed

Gorse – they lack faith in their success or improvement, and are convinced they will not succeed, so give up

Hornbeam – they lack the mental and physical strength to do the tasks ahead of them, often putting things off

Scleranthus – they are not sure if they will make the right decision, whether it is a big decision or just a trivial matter, but still they do not ask others for advice

Wild Oat – they are insecure when it comes to choosing a life direction when they are at a crossroads

DISTRIBUTION AND APPLICATION OF BACH FLOWER REMEDIES IN THE WORLD

Today, Bach flower remedies are very famous and widespread in the world. They are usually sold in pharmacies and in stores specialising in the sale of natural products. They are registered and accepted in almost all countries of the European Union, and are sold worldwide. The combination of five flower remedies, known as 'the crisis mix', is produced by many makers under different brand names and has been tried by many people in times of stress.

There are currently more than 3,000[2] active Bach Flower Registered Practitioners worldwide, in more than 70 countries.[3] There are still far more people who use Bach flower remedies for their personal needs, by layman's choice, just

---

[2] https://www.bachcentre.com/new/en/contact/practitioners/, Register of Active Bach Foundation Registered Practitioners, as of 19 July 2020.

[3] The Bach Centre Register lists the areas of the United Kingdom separately: England, Wales, Scotland, Northern Ireland and the Isle of Man.

ıs Dr. Bach envisioned – that every household would have a set of Bach flower remedies at home and that they would choose which flower remedies they needed at a particular moment.

Bach's texts have been translated into many different languages, and education about this system is conducted around the world by local teachers approved by The Bach Centre.

ABOUT EDWARD BACH

Dr. Edward Bach was born on 24 September 1886, in the town of Moseley, not far from Birmingham. He studied medicine at Birmingham University and later at University College Hospital in London, where in 1912 he graduated and continued to work as a surgeon. He later worked as a bacteriologist and pathologist, and undertook various researches on vaccines in his laboratory. In 1919 he went to work at the London Homeopathic Hospital, where he began to study homeopathy, resulting in the discovery of seven homeopathic nosodes, which are still in use today. He regularly published the results of his research in professional journals such as the *British Homeopathic Journal*, *Medical World* and *Homeopathic World*. He discovered a new system of treatment with flower remedies in 1928, when he discovered the first plants: Impatiens, Mimulus and Clematis. Then he stopped using nosodes and started working on a system of simple healing treatment with flower remedies. In 1930 he left London and his work as a doctor, and went out in nature, in search of medicinal plants. He moved to Mount Vernon – a house in Brightwell-cum-Sotwell, Oxfordshire – in 1934, and spent the last years of his life there. There he found the last 19 plants and completed the system of 38 flower remedies.

He died on 27 November 1936, shortly after publishing his most significant work, *The Twelve Healers and Other Remedies*, in which he described his discoveries – 38 flower remedies and the methods of their preparation: the *sunshine method* and the *boiling method*. He passed on his work to his assistants, Nora Weeks and Victor Bullen, who continued to teach and spread Dr. Bach's method of healing with flower remedies, and founded The Bach Centre in Mount Vernon house.

ABOUT THE BACH CENTRE

The Bach Centre is located in Mount Vernon house, in the village of Brightwell-cum-Sotwell, not far from the outskirts of London. There you will find the house in which Dr. Edward Bach spent the last few years of his life and the garden in which you may see many of the plants from Dr. Bach's flower remedies system. The Bach Centre was founded by Dr. Bach's closest associates, Nora Weeks and Victor Bullen, who were personally trained by Dr. Bach in how to prepare flower remedies.

There is a plate on the door of The Bach Centre that reads: 'SIMPLICITY – HUMILITY – COMPASSION', which represents Dr. Bach's deepest beliefs and describes his system. Today, The Bach Centre organises education on Bach flower remedies, and even now flower remedies are prepared in the garden according to the principles of Dr. Bach.

At the Centre you can see Dr. Bach's room, where he held his consultations, the furniture he personally made, and his original mother tinctures. A large number of plants from which flower remedies are made grow in the garden, the preparation of which you can observe if you are lucky, during your visit to The Bach Centre on a sunny day.

Judy Ramsell Howard is a trustee of the Dr. Edward Bach Healing Trust, which owns Mount Vernon house. Judy is the daughter of John Ramsell, to whom Dr. Bach's method was personally passed on by Nora Weeks and Victor Bullen. Judy is also a Director of the Bach Visitor and Education Centre, as is Stefan Ball. The team of people at The Bach Centre still cherish the values established by Dr. Edward Bach, and their primary concern is that the Bach flower remedies system maintains the simplicity requested by Dr. Bach. The Bach Centre has always been passed down, with each generation promising to maintain the system of Bach flower remedies in line with the principles set by Dr. Bach.

Thus, the transfer of knowledge and values about Dr. Bach's flower remedies has been performed several times so far, always with a promise made to Dr. Bach and the system by the persons chosen to continue and nurture the system further into the future:

1. Dr. Edward Bach passed the system on to his close associates, Nora Weeks and Victor Bullen. They founded The Bach Centre after Dr. Bach's death, in the house where Dr. Bach spent the last years of his life.

1. Victor Bullen died in 1975, and Nora Weeks in 1978. Nora Weeks transferred The Bach Centre to Nickie Murray and her brother John Ramsell, who had been associates at the Centre since the 1960s.

2. John Ramsell passed on his knowledge and Dr. Bach's values to his daughter Judy Ramsell Howard, who joined the team in 1985 and who now runs The Bach Centre.

Stefan Ball, like Judy, has also sworn to maintain The Bach Centre and system and, among other things, oversees training and maintains the Bach Foundation International Register of Practitioners. Today, Judy's children – her son Sam and her daughter Fay – also work at The Bach Centre. It is to be expected that Bach's legacy will continue to be passed on in the same way to younger generations.

At The Bach Centre, you still feel that positive atmosphere when you walk through the house and garden where Dr. Bach worked on the discovery of the flower remedies and where he spent the last few years of his life. That is why today The Bach Centre is visited by people from all parts of the world, in search of knowledge, plants, peace and health.

DR. BACH'S WRITINGS AND THE DEVELOPMENT OF THE SYSTEM OVER TIME

Dr. Edward Bach began his professional life as an employee in a family business, but it became clear to him the very first day that he did not belong there. He wanted to be a doctor and help others. Thus, at the age of 20 he left that job and enrolled in medical school at the University of Birmingham.

He received his medical degree in 1912 (Diploma of Public Health) from the University Hospital in Cambridge.

In 1919, Dr. Bach started working as a homeopathic doctor at the Royal London Homeopathic Hospital. Today the hospital operates under the name Royal London Hospital for Integrated Medicine, its title having been changed to reflect the fact that the hospital practises other methods of treatment as well as homeopathy.

At the time, being an employee at the Royal London Homeopathic Hospital was a prestigious job for Dr. Bach. Throughout its history, apart from Dr. Bach, other famous homeopaths, like John Henry Clarke and Margaret Tyler, among others, have worked in this hospital.

The hospital was founded in 1849 by Dr. Frederick Foster Harvey Quinn, who was one of the first physicians to practise homeopathy in England, and learned about homeopathy from Samuel Hahnemann himself. Dr. Quinn was a prominent figure in London's social circles because he was the personal physician and homeopath of Prince Leopold, the father-in-law of Queen Victoria and father of Prince Albert. He was a very good friend of Charles Dickens and a godfather to his child.

In the period when Dr. Bach was working at that hospital, it gained the patronage of His Highness the Duke of York, who later became King George VI. From 1947 up to the present day, the hospital has been called 'Royal', to indicate that it is under royal patronage. Today, Queen Elizabeth II is patron of the hospital.

During his work at the hospital, Dr. Bach made numerous contributions to medicine and homeopathy. As a homeopath, he discovered seven types of homeopathic nosodes that are still used in homeopathic practice today. These nosodes were used in his time by homeopaths and doctors in England, Germany and America. Because of his contributions to homeopathy, other homeopaths called him 'the second Hahnemann',[4] in particular because, like Dr. Hahnemann, he wrote mostly about chronic diseases.

He also published some of the most relevant papers on medicine and homeopathy of the period, between 1920 and 1930:

- 'The relation of vaccine therapy to homeopathy', *British Homeopathic Journal*, April 1920.

- 'The problem of chronic disease', *International Homeopathy Congress*, London, 1924.

- 'A note on vaccines potentized', *British Homeopathic Journal*, 1927.

- 'An effective way of combating intestinal toxaemia', *Medical World*, London, 1928.

- 'Rediscovery of psora', *British Homeopathic Journal*, January 1929.

- 'Intestinal nosodes', *British Homeopathic Journal*, 1930.

- 'Medicine of the future', *Homeopathic World*, February 1930.

- 'Some fundamental considerations of disease and cure', *Homeopathic World*, October 1930.

- 'An effective method of preparing vaccines for oral administration', *Medical World*, January 1930.

Although at first it seemed that classical medicine was his real calling and occupation, he again felt dissatisfaction because he realised that he was not helping his patients enough. Dr. Bach spent hours and hours sitting next to his

---

[4]   Dr. Samuel Hahnemann was the founder of homeopathy. Source: Nora Weeks, The Medical Discoveries of Edward Bach, Physician, The C.W. Daniel Company Limited (1975), p. 32.

patients and listening to their ailments, trying to puzzle out the cause of their illnesses. This motivation stayed with him until the end of his life – that desire to help patients eliminate the root cause of their diseases. He believed that it was his life's calling to discover a simple system of natural healing treatments that people around the world would be able to use on their own.

Dr. Edward Bach published his first observations on medicinal plants in the February 1930 issue of *Homeopathic World*, under the title 'Some new remedies and new uses'. In this paper he described five medicinal plants, three of which are plants from the present-day system of Bach flower remedies: Impatiens, Mimulus and Clematis. However, as Dr. Bach was both a physician and a homeopath, he established those first works on the basis of these plants' healing properties, by applying homeopathic principles; hence he prepared them as homeopathic remedies and not as flower remedies.

His deepest longing — to discover a system of natural healing available to all — led him in the exact opposite direction from the one that was expected of him. Instead of continuing to build his successful medical career, to the astonishment of his colleagues and to the disappointment of his then-patients, he left his job in London and went out into nature in search of medicinal plants. He was certain that the Divine gift in nature provided the cure for all our human afflictions and sufferings. He believed that all diseases disappear when we are happy and attuned to our soul and when we do the work we are destined to do by birth. He sought medicines that would alleviate the fears and sufferings of the sick, and strengthen their intention to heal. So in 1930 Dr. Bach left his job as a physician and set out to search for medicines in nature.

By 1932, Dr. Bach had discovered twelve flower remedies, which he described in a booklet entitled *Free Thyself*.

In the spring of 1933, he published two articles: 'Twelve great remedies' and 'Twelve healers'.

These twelve healers were as follows:

1. CHICORY *(Cichorium intybus)*
2. MIMULUS *(Mimulus luteus)*
3. AGRIMONY *(Agrimonia eupatoria)*
4. SCLERANTHUS *(Scleranthus annuus)*
5. CLEMATIS *(Clematis vitalba)*
6. CENTAURY *(Erythraea centaurium)*
7. GENTIAN *(Gentiana amarella)*
8. VERVAIN *(Verbena officinalis)*
9. CERATO *(Ceratostigma willmottiana)*
10. IMPATIENS *(Impatiens royleii)*
11. ROCK ROSE *(Helianthemum vulgare)*
12. WATER VIOLET (*Hottonia palustris*)

In the autumn of 1933, Bach expanded the system with four new remedies and published the book *The Twelve Healers and Four Helpers*.

The four helpers were the following plants, or remedies:

1. GORSE (*Ulex europaeus*)
2. OAK (*Quercus pedunculata*)[5]
3. HEATHER (*Calluna vulgaris*)
4. ROCK WATER (spring water with medicinal properties)

---

[5] Modern name: *Quercus robur.*

In 1934, he described the four helpers in *The Story of the Zodiac* as follows: 'The Four Helpers were the faith in a better world which they hoped one day to attain, now reflected in the flaming Gorse bush. The perseverance of the Oak which braved all tempests, offering shelter and support to the weaker things. The willingness to serve of Heather, which was glad to cover with its simple beauty the arid wind-tossed spaces, and the pure springs gushing from the rocks, bringing brightness and refreshment to those weary and sore after battle.'

In 1934, Dr. Bach moved in to Mount Vernon, the house now known as The Bach Centre. His assistants, Nora Weeks (1896–1978) and Victor Bullen (1887–1975), worked alongside him on the team, as did Mary Tabor, who left the team sometime during the 1940s and wrote her novel *To Thine Own Self*, in which details from the life and work of Dr. Bach and his team can be recognised, although the novel is fiction.

In July 1934, Dr. Bach published the second edition of his book, which contained three additional flower remedies – Olive, Vine and Wild Oat – and was published under the new title *The Twelve Healers and Seven Helpers*.

These seven helpers were:

1. GORSE (*Ulex europaeus*)
2. OAK (*Quercus pedunculata*)
3. HEATHER (*Calluna vulgaris*)
4. ROCK WATER (spring water with medicinal properties)
5. OLIVE (*Olea europaea*)
6. VINE (*Vitis vinifera*)
7. WILD OAT (*Bromus asper*)[6]

---

[6]   Modern name: *Bromus ramosus*.

By the autumn of 1935, Dr. Bach had discovered nine-teen new flower remedies, as well as the boiling method of preparing remedies. Information about these new remedies was printed in the form of a leaflet, which was inserted into the remaining stock of the book *Twelve healers and seven helpers.*

On Dr. Bach's 50th birthday, 24 September 1936, the book *The Twelve Healers and Other Remedies* was published.

The final list containing all 38 remedies is stated in that book as shown in Table 2.[7]

Table 2. *The final list of all 38 remedies as published in* The Twelve Healers and Other Remedies

BACH FLOWER REMEDIES	LATIN NAME OF THE PLANT
Agrimony*	*Agrimonia Eupatoria*
Aspen	*Populus Tremula*
Beech	*Fagus Sylvatica*
Centaury*	*Erythraea Centaurium*
Cerato*	*Ceratostigma Willmottiana*
Cherry Plum	*Prunus Cerasifera*
Chestnut Bud	*Aesculus Hippocastanum*
Chicory*	*Cichorium Intybus*
Clematis*	*Clematis Vitalba*
Crab Apple	*Pyrus Malus*
Elm	*Ulmus Campestris*

---

[7] Contrary to Bach's wishes, the publisher marked in the book the twelve flower essences which were originally called 'twelve healers' with asterisks, so that readers would have the information about the twelve essences listed in the title of the book. Readers were already used to that title of the book, so the publisher wanted to retain that recognisable title. Here I present a list of the essences as they were originally listed in that book.

Gentian*	Gentiana Amarella
Gorse	Ulex Europaeus
Heather	Calluna Vulgaris
Holly	Ilex Aquifolium
Honeysuckle	Lonicera Caprifolium
Hornbeam	Carpinus Betulus
Impatiens*	Impatiens Royleii
Larch	Larix Europaea
Mimulus*	Mimulus Luteus
Mustard	Sinapis Arvensis
Oak	Quercus Pedunculata
Olive	Olea Europaea
Pine	Pinus Sylvestris
Red Chestnut	Aesculus Carnea
Rock Rose*	Helianthemum Vulgare
Rock Water	Spring water
Scleranthus*	Scleranthus Annuus
Star of Bethlehem	Ornithogalum Umbellatum
Sweet Chestnut	Castanea Vulgaris
Vervain*	Verbena Officinalis
Vine	Vitis Vinifera
Walnut	Juglans Regia
Water Violet*	Hottonia Palustris
White Chestnut	Aesculus Hippocastanum
Wild Oat	Bromus Asper
Wild Rose	Rosa Canina
Willow	Salix Vitellina

Note: As in Table 1, earlier in the book, I have retained Dr. Bach's usage here, which is to present plants' Latin names with an initial capital on the second word as well as the first.

On 27 November 1936, Dr. Edward Bach died in his sleep. He passed away very soon after concluding his research and handing the system over to his students, Nora Weeks and Victor Bullen. They continued to spread the teachings of Dr. Bach, and the same is being done very successfully today by the staff of The Bach Centre in the small, beautiful village of Brightwell-cum-Sotwell, South Oxfordshire.

The last edition, which is considered the final version of the book, was published in 1941, and contains a longer introduction dictated by Dr. Bach to his assistant, Nora Weeks, on 30 October 1936, as one of his last works in life.

The book *Twelve Healers and Other Remedies* has been published continuously since then. It has been translated into most of the world's major languages, in Croatian as well, and has been published in countless editions. Over the years, the original descriptions of the flower remedies have remained identical to those described by Dr. Edward Bach.

In this book you are reading, the original description for each flower remedy is specified in Part Two of the book, as taken from that final edition. Descriptions of the flowers or some interesting facts about the remedies are also included in this book, as taken from the biographies and works of Dr. Bach.

For each essence mentioned in this book, it is stated which flower remedies had been defined by Dr. Bach as a type, and which represent only the state of mind into which a person falls due to external circumstances. Each remedy can be taken for a state of mind, and only some of the remedies from the system represent a personality type. Dr. Bach did not leave a definitive list of flower remedies that represent a type, so for some flower remedies we can only discuss whether such flower remedies can represent a person's type.

As I mentioned previously, the historical development of the system, with a '12/7/19' distinction of the remedies, where Dr. Bach started the system with the first twelve remedies known as the 'twelve healers', followed by adding seven new remedies known as the 'seven helpers', and expanded even further with another nineteen new remedies, it might be helpful for your studies to make the point here clearly that <u>this distinction was abandoned in the final system</u>. The reason for this is as follows: in part because the remedies didn't fit well in those boxes of 'healers' and 'helpers', and in part because, in practice, these distinctions weren't useful when it came to selecting remedies. Therefore, today we have a system of 38 flower remedies, and we don't need to group them into healers and helpers. The only reason I mention these in this book is so that readers can be familiar with the historical development of the system.

BASIC CHARACTERISTICS OF THE BACH FLOWER REMEDIES SYSTEM

Dr. Edward Bach described the system of Bach flower remedies as follows:

'The main principles are these:

Firstly. That no medical knowledge whatever is required.

Secondly. That the disease itself is of no consequence whatsoever.

Thirdly. That the mind is the most sensitive part of our bodies, and hence the best guide to tell us what remedy is required.

Fourthly. Thus the manner in which a patient reacts to an illness is alone taken into account. Not the illness itself.

Fifthly. That such as: fear, depression, doubt, hopelessness, irritability, desire for company or desire to be alone, indecision, such are the true guides to the way in which a patient is being affected by his malady, and to the Remedy which he needs.'

Furthermore, Dr. Bach explains the advantages of this healing method over other methods of treatment:

'The system being spoken of this evening has great advantages over others.

Firstly. All the remedies are made from beautiful flowers, plants and trees of Nature: none of them are poisonous nor can do any harm, no matter how much was taken.

Secondly. They are only 38 in number, which means that it is easier to find the right herb to give, than when there are very many.

Thirdly. The method of choosing which remedies to give is simple enough for most people to understand.

Fourthly. The cures which have been obtained have been so wonderful, that they have passed all expectations of even those who use this method, as well as the patients who have received the benefit.

These herbs have succeeded again and again where all other treatment, which has been tried, has failed.'

Edward Bach, 1936

The above features are given, I believe, in comparison with the homeopathy practised by Dr. Bach. In homeopathy, some poisonous[8] plants, minerals and animal secretions are used as sources in the preparation of homeopathic remedies. Additionally in homeopathy, a homeopathic remedy's potency during its preparation is also important, which is not the case with Bach flower remedies. Today, homeopaths can use more than five thousand homeopathic remedies in their practice, which is much more demanding to study and work

---

[8] Safe for use when prepared in homeopathic form.

with when compared to Bach flower remedies. Homeopathy is a complex system requiring many years of study, which are of crucial importance if a person is to become able to apply the system independently; while Dr. Bach sought to devise a system that could be used independently by each member of a household, regardless of their education and age.

Dr. Bach, according to Nora Weeks, felt that 'The right remedies would cause no severe reactions, neither would they be harmful or unpleasant to take; their effect would be gentle and sure, resulting in a healing of both body and mind.'[9]

As a guide to physicians, homeopaths and other therapists, and especially to those who will apply Bach flower remedies as a healing method in their work, Dr. Bach provided clear instructions on how to talk to patients:

'... never allow patients to talk about the past. The illness of yesterday is of yesterday, and of no interest or importance now. What we have to treat is the present state of the patient, exactly as he is at the time we see him, and even when we see him again in a further week, he is again a new patient. Improvements may have occurred and alterations taken place, which now mean that he may require another remedy, and even the interval of a week gone by is past history and of no present consequence. In acute cases our patient may be a new man, a different case within a few hours. We must ever treat the present NOW, and to think back or to allow a patient to dwell on the past is hampering in its results.'[10]

To summarise, the system of Bach flower remedies is:

9   Nora Weeks, The Medical Discoveries of Edward Bach, Physician, The C.W. Daniel Company Limited (1975), p. 48.
10   Bach, E., Two More Essentials, The Bach Centre (2014).

- ✓ Simple
- ✓ Natural
- ✓ Suitable for home use
- ✓ Complementary with all other therapies
- ✓ There are no consequences from 'wrongly' selected remedies
- ✓ No addiction is possible
- ✓ No overdose
- ✓ No side effects
- ✓ Safe for babies and pregnant women

EFFECTS OF FLOWER REMEDIES

Flower remedies do not change the chemical composition of our body and are not substances dangerous for our body. They encourage the development of the positive qualities we already possess, and restore our balance and health. But bear in mind that remedies cannot develop in us some quality that we do not already possess. There are no dramatic negative effects during the application of the remedies. Acute situations are resolved instantly, and long-term problems take a little longer. Each person reacts differently, and the effect of peeling back the layers will be the same as peeling onions – only one layer at a time is cleaned.

METHODS
OF PREPARATION

Two methods are used for the preparation of Bach flower remedies: the sunshine method and the boiling method. These are described below.

THE SUNSHINE METHOD

Dr. Bach describes the sunshine method with these words:

'A thin glass bowl is taken and almost filled with the purest water obtainable, if possible from a spring nearby.

The blooms of the plant are picked and immediately floated on the surface of the water, so as to cover it, and then left in the bright sunshine for three or four hours, or less time if the blooms begin to show signs of fading. The blossoms are then carefully lifted out and the water poured into bottles so as to half fill them. The bottles are then filled up with brandy to preserve the remedy. These bottles are stock, and are not used direct for giving doses. A few flower essences are taken from these to another bottle, from which the patient is treated, so that the stocks contain a large supply …'.

The following remedies are prepared using the sunshine method: Agrimony, Centaury, Cerato, Chicory, Clematis, Gentian, Gorse, Heather, Impatiens, Mimulus, Oak, Olive, Rock Rose, Rock Water, Scleranthus, Wild Oat, Vervain, Vine, Water Violet, White Chestnut Blossom.

Rock Water is the only remedy in the system that is not prepared from flowers. Dr. Bach explained the use of rock water with these words: 'It has long been known that certain wells and spring waters have had the power to heal some people, and such wells or springs have become renowned for this property. Any well or any spring which has been known to have had healing power and which is still left free in its natural state, unhampered by the shrines of man, may be used.'

THE BOILING METHOD

The remaining remedies are prepared by the boiling method. Dr. Bach came to the idea of applying this method to those flowers that blossomed in the spring or autumn, when the sun was not so strong, meaning he could not use the energy of the sun in the preparation of the remedies. The first remedy prepared using the boiling method was Cherry Plum.

'The specimens, as about to be described, were boiled for half an hour in clean pure water. The rest of the procedure is the same. The fluid strained off, poured into bottles until half filled, and then, when cold, brandy added as before to fill up and preserve.'

The following remedies are prepared with the boiling method: Aspen, Beech, Cherry Plum, Chestnut Bud, Crab Apple, Elm, Holly, Honeysuckle, Hornbeam, Larch, Mustard, Pine, Red Chestnut, Star of Bethlehem, Sweet Chestnut, Walnut, Wild Rose, Willow.

The blossom should be used together with small pieces of stem or stalk and, when present, young fresh leaves. One exception to this rule is Chestnut Bud. For this remedy the buds are gathered from the White Chestnut tree, just before it bursts into leaf.

INTERESTING FACT

All of these plants can be found growing in nature on the British Isles, with the exception of Vine, Olive and Cerato, although some of them originated directly from other countries throughout central and northern Europe, all the way to northern India and Tibet.

Cerato originally grew in Tibet, in the land of wisdom and spirituality, so it is not surprising that the basic function of these flower remedies is to strengthen intuition.

The flower remedies of Olive and Vine were prepared for Dr. Bach by his friends from Italy and Switzerland. Thus, the parent tinctures of Vine and Olive were prepared by the method of sun exposure in Italy, while the remedy of Vine was prepared by the same method in Switzerland.

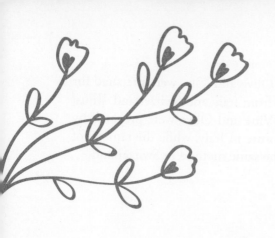

PART TWO

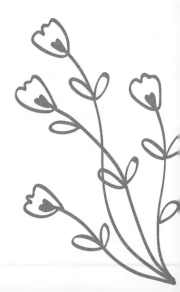

PART TWO

Bach flower remedies: 38 flower remedies

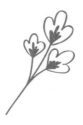

AGRIMONY
Agrimonia eupatoria

Dr. Bach's description of the flower: '… beautiful plant Agrimony, growing along the sides of our lanes and in our meadows, with its church-like spire, and its seeds like bells …'

Dr. Bach's final description of the flower remedy: 'The jovial, cheerful, humorous people who love peace and are distressed by argument or quarrel, to avoid which they will agree to give up much. Though generally they have troubles and are tormented and restless and worried in mind or in body, they hide their cares behind their humour and jesting and are considered very good friends to know. They often take alcohol or drugs in excess, to stimulate and help themselves bear their trials with cheerfulness.'

Description from *The Story of the Travellers* **(1934):** Indication: 'Agrimony began to be worried ...' Positive outcome: 'Agrimony strides along free of all care, and jests on everything.'

Group of remedies: for those over-sensitive to influences and ideas

Key words for recognising the remedy: mask, escape from problems, hiding problems

Common expressions: to the question 'How are you?' the person will reply briefly: 'I am fine, everything is well, everything is fine, never better.' They joke at their own expense. They use jokes, proverbs, sayings and counter-questions in response to delicate questions about themselves and their problems.

Personality type: a fun and cheerful person, a social butterfly loved in society, but can also be a person prone to vices. A person who runs away from problems into alcohol, drugs, entertainment, other vices. They escape from the problem by staying away from home, so as not to face their own thoughts. They run away from problems into fun, all with the goal of being away from home. You will recognise that person by their smile and cheerful face, despite the problems, while often it is just a fake smile, because they do not show their flaws, problems or bad mood in front of others, and pretend to be well.

Examples of situations where we might consider this remedy: a situation in which the person should present themselves in public in a good light. Examples of such conditions:

- A husband and wife quarrelled just before going out to dinner with friends. At dinner, they will act as if nothing had happened, even though they know that it troubles them. As long as they are at the dinner, they will laugh and have fun. When they get home, then they can take off their masks and may continue to quarrel or not communicate with each other at all.

- Graduation anniversary, where a person wants to present only their best self, and hides their failures or problems behind a smile or a joke.

- A person has just lost a lot of money gambling and cannot share their worries with their family who do not know about their vice. They come home and pretend that everything is fine, even though the problem troubles them.

- The person goes to hang out with friends and does not want to show their worry about the problems they are experiencing. They will be in a cheerful mood at the gathering and will hide their problems behind a smile.

Examples of people who might need this flower remedy: because of the role they are asked to play in public, public figures might be especially prone to adopting an Agrimony mask, like members of the royal family, public figures, actors; but also all other 'ordinary' people might need Agrimony too, if they do not wish to show their true feelings or problems in front of others.

Positive outcome of the application of this flower remedy: a person will realise that they will not be rejected by others if they show their weaknesses, problems or worries in front of them. They will no longer bear the burden of their problems alone, like some dark secret, but will be able to open up to others and talk about their problems or shortcomings.

Note: these are not standard or the only flower remedies for quitting drinking or other addictions, nor are these flower remedies intended exclusively for people who have such addictions. It is possible for a person to be an Agrimony type without consuming alcohol at all, or having any other vices. An essential characteristic for choosing this flower remedy is that the person hides their worries and problems behind a cheerful face and does not allow others to grasp their problems.

EXAMPLES FROM PRACTICE

In my introductory story at the beginning of the book, I stated that Agrimony flower remedy was in the first Bach flower remedies bottle I took. I was an Agrimony person at the time. At least that is how I thought of myself then. Today I see that I was not an Agrimony type, but I was just taught to behave that way, which was not my true nature. My real personality is something quite the opposite of Agrimony, considering I had never drunk, smoked or partied. But I really possessed the most important characteristic of the Agrimony flower remedy – hiding my worries behind a smiling face. I was actually taught to behave like that from a young age. My parents taught me that problems and difficulties are never to be vented outside the house. I was clearly instructed that, on the outside, the family should always look perfect. And that is how I obediently behaved for years. It was especially important to withhold information about a bad grade (yes, I also had Fs), and one of the most important things was to wipe the dust every day in case some guests came unannounced. Today I see that these were all instructions that were aimed at creating an image of perfection in every aspect, while hiding anything remotely negative.

And what happened when I took my first bottle of flower remedies with Agrimony in it? I very quickly rejected the rules I had learned. I realised that nothing would happen if someone heard about some of my flaws or omissions, or my real stories. And that was the point at which I basically discovered my ability to work with people. Because it is impossible to work with people who have problems without at some point sharing some of the difficulties you have been through and that you have overcome, as a sign of encouragement and inspiration to clients, so they can see that problems can be surmounted. This book would never have been written if I hadn't taken Agrimony flower remedy.

Here I also cite the example of a person who is a true Agrimony type: a merry man, a favourite in social circles, always replying to all questions with jokes and witty stories. He liked company, fun, a glass or two of alcohol (or ten). He listened to the problems of others, but did not talk about his own. He turned to me for help as he was going through marital problems. It was amazing that one bottle of flower remedies completely transformed him. Today he is a completely different person. Although he is still basically an Agrimony type, who is cheerful and a favourite of society, the negative sides of the Agrimony type are balanced. Today, he is a counsellor himself, working with people and helping them to overcome life crises. His experiences prompted him to focus his practice on helping others. In his work, he openly talks about the life difficulties that he overcame.

But while these two stories suggest that individuals eventually become counsellors to others, this may not always be the outcome of the application of the remedies. After a person takes this flower remedy, they will realise that sometimes it is natural to share their problems with others. And they will be able to open up to dear people they trust, instead of escaping into the world of entertainment and alcohol.

Here I want to compare the Agrimony flower remedy with other flower remedies:

- Agrimony can be prone to vices and alcohol, unlike Rock Water who has exceptional self-discipline and is less susceptible to vices.

- Agrimony does not talk about their problems, unlike Heather who tells them to everyone.

- Although both Agrimony and Water Violet do not like to talk about their problems with others, Agrimony loves company and is an extroverted type, unlike Water Violet who is a loner and loves solitude.

 Remember: Agrimony wears a mask of a cheerful and smiling face and will never show their emotions in company. This flower remedy help us take off the weight of that mask, so that we can open up to others and share our worries, instead of escaping into a world of fun and vice.

ASPEN

Populus tremula

Dr. Bach's final description of the flower remedy: 'Vague unknown fears, for which there can be given no explanation, no reason. Yet the patient may be terrified of something terrible going to happen, he knows not what. These vague unexplainable fears may haunt by night or day. Sufferers often are afraid to tell their trouble to others.'

Dr. Bach's lecture on this flower remedy: 'The third kind of fear is of those vague unaccountable things which cannot be explained. As if something dreadful is going to happen, without any idea as to what it may be. All such dreads for which no reason can be given, and yet are very real and disturbing to the individual, require the Remedy of the ASPEN TREE. And the relief which this has brought to many is truly wonderful.'

Group of remedies: for fear

Key words for recognising the remedy: unknown fear, fear with no apparent cause

Common expressions: 'I have a bad feeling that something could happen', 'I feel that something is wrong', 'it is acted upon by some invisible forces', 'This house feels like it is haunted.'

State of mind or personality type: Dr. Bach did not define Aspen flower remedy as a definite type of person. This is one of those remedies that belongs to the so-called grey zone when choosing the type of remedy for a person. A person who could be an Aspen type is full of fears related to invisible spheres – they are sensitive to all 'invisible' stimuli from the environment – but in practice, Aspen would be seen more as a state-of-mind remedy, and not a type.

Examples of situations where we might consider this remedy: situations in which a person feels the fear, but without some specific cause, as it is more of an undefined fear or a hunch that something bad might happen.

Examples of people who might need this flower remedy: anyone who is afraid and cannot say why, and cannot name the fear.

Difference between Aspen, Mimulus and Rock Rose fear:

Mimulus is the remedy for known fears – fears that we can explain and give a name. If we can name the fear it is a known fear, even if the cause of the fear is fictional or uncanny. Mimulus is the right remedy to consider in this situation.

Aspen should be used when we don't know why we are afraid.

A boy can be frightened because he's seen ghosts on a TV programme, and this is a Mimulus state, as he knows what he is afraid of.

An Aspen state is when a boy goes into a building and feel there is something weird and wrong about it, but can't say what. He will not say that he is afraid of ghosts, but he will say that he feels uncomfortable in this building, but doesn't know why.

Both types of fear, Aspen and Mimulus, can grow into a more powerful extreme type of fear – Rock Rose, which represents panic fear – whether of a known or unknown cause.

Positive outcome of the application of this flower remedy: Positive outcome is a not to be afraid when there is nothing to be afraid of.

EXAMPLES FROM PRACTICE

Once a seven-year-old boy was brought for consultations who was completely in a state of Aspen flower remedy. He was afraid to sleep alone or be alone in a room because, he said, he felt some negative forces that scared him. After two bottles of flower remedies, he told me he could still sense these bad forces, but he was no longer afraid of them.

One client, on the other hand, was dreadfully afraid that something terrible might happen when she was home alone in the evening, but she could not determine what. She was not afraid of thieves or darkness, but simply felt uneasy. She could not fall asleep because she had a feeling, late into the night, that something awful could happen if she fell asleep. Only two days after she started taking Aspen flower remedy, she was able to fall asleep normally and no longer had that uncomfortable feeling. She continued to take these flower remedies for a few more months because she felt they gave her security and calmness.

 Remember: Aspen helps when we are afraid and we don't know why we are afraid. This flower remedy will give us the courage to face uncomfortable situations and places, when we feel fear without the proper cause or without being able to name it.

BEECH

Fagus sylvatica

Dr. Bach's final description of the flower remedy: 'For those who feel the need to see more good and beauty in all that surrounds them. And, although much appears to be wrong, to have the ability to see the good growing within. So as to be able to be more tolerant, lenient and understanding of the different way each individual and all things are working to their own final perfection.'

Group of remedies: for over-care for welfare of others

Key words for recognising the remedy: criticism, intolerance and pointing out of other people's flaws, omissions, actions, appearance, traits, choice of partner or occupation, etc.

Common expressions: 'How can you do that?', 'Look at yourself!', 'Get a hold of yourself!', 'Did you gain weight?'

Personality type: a person who constantly criticises, points out others' omissions and flaws. The person has an attitude as if they are the ones doing things best, as if they know best, or as if they are already an example of perfection. Beech responds to other people's attitudes, actions or looks, and certain people will get on their nerves, they will roll their eyes and find it difficult to refrain from criticism.

Examples of situations where we might consider this remedy: a situation in which a person faces other people's flaws, stances or actions, during family gatherings, at work, in society.

Examples of people who might need this flower remedy: anyone who is prone to criticising others, has no tolerance for the flaws and behaviour of others, directs criticism without restraint, and gives unsolicited advice on how a person can improve themselves or what they are doing.

Positive outcome of the application of this flower remedy: Dr. Bach himself illustrated the positive outcome of this flower remedy in its description and did not focus on the negative aspects. According to Dr. Bach, a person will see more good and beautiful things in everything that surrounds them after taking Beech flower remedy. Instead of focusing on everything that is wrong, the person will see what is positive. The person will become more tolerant, more lenient and will have more understanding for the different ways each individual does things. A person will let others make their own decisions and live their choices, without interference. They will give advice only when the other person asks for it.

Tip for Beech types: when you want to give advice, you don't need to do so in the form of a command or instruction, but it is possible to start a sentence in the following manner: 'In your place, I would do this or that, but you do as you think is best for you ...'. Even though, in many situations, such a sentence would not sound critical, Stefan Ball says[11] that 'there's a good chance that a person in a true Beech state saying those words is still going to sound very critical and interfering.' So, the tone of voice and intention needs to be considered too while saying these things, if you don't want to sound critical or intrusive.

And, second, if you were not asked for your advice or opinion, do not express it; your interlocutor could be offended. They will not see it as benevolent advice or comment, but as interference and malice. Therefore, wait until you are asked for your advice or opinion before expressing it. If they don't ask you, let them solve their problems on their own. Just let them know you're there for them if they need you.

The difference between a Beech and a Rock Water personality type: Beech believes that they do everything perfectly and that they themselves are an example of perfection, so they want to align other people with themselves, for their own good. They do this through criticism, giving unsolicited advice, through comments, sarcasm, etc. Rock Water also believes they are an example of perfection in everything they do, but do not impose their opinion on others, nor criticise, nor give advice. Instead, they hope others will notice their

---

[11]   Correspondence via e-mail on the topic of Beech flower remedy.

virtues and qualities, way of working or lifestyle, and will want to follow their example.

EXAMPLES FROM PRACTICE

That a Beech person cannot refrain from comments and criticism I was convinced many times in my life. Here I will give two examples of a Beech person that I often talk about in seminars when I am trying to portray a Beech person. I give these two examples because they are typical of Beech – the criticism in these stories was directed at me, and in both cases the person tried to point out to me with a comment what I was doing wrong, although I had neither sought nor expected advice.

On one occasion I had a client in for a consultation, who told me about her difficult personal problems. That was our second meeting and I had known the client for only a short period of time. She was telling me her sad life story and was trying to portray herself and the other persons in that story. She was describing herself, talking about what kind of person she was and what her characteristics were. And that is how she came to utter the following sentence: 'You know, I am a very honest person. What I think of someone, I say without hesitation. So, for example, if, when I come to see you for consultations, you put on this striped dress, and you also put on this scarf with butterflies, which never match, then I will openly tell you that. I will tell you: "This combination is really not congruent; but, maybe you are happy with these butterflies, so I will let it be."'

So, in the middle of a very serious story, which was really very dramatic, when I was one hundred per cent focused on the consultation, I suddenly heard the unexpected – criticism of the outfit I had chosen to wear that day – and I thought to myself, 'Is it possible that she has just criticised me?!' And in an instant I was surprised and confused, and then I laughed. And I realised that in front of me was a typical Beech person, who could not help herself, despite the fact that I was the person who was helping her and who was her advisor, and to whom she came for help – she could not help herself, because she thought that the advice would help me not to repeat the mistake and wear such an 'incompatible' clothing combination again in the future.

The second example is similar – I also received criticism when I least expected it, without seeking advice, from a person who does not even know me.

Before one seminar I had organised at my centre, I went to the store and bought twelve donuts. I planned to serve the donuts with snacks, coffee and tea to the seminar participants during a break. When it was my turn at the checkout, the cashier asked me, 'Why do you need so many donuts?' I told her that I had a seminar today and that I had bought them for the students. She answered me: 'For God's sake, don't you have anything healthier to feed your clients?! Why did you buy donuts for these people? Serve them something healthier.' And in this situation, I was astounded by the comment of an unknown person, who had just reprimanded me and condemned my choice of sweets for my clients. I paid for the donuts, served them to the clients, and since then I have always told this amusing story during seminar breaks.

Of these two well-meaning unsolicited pieces of advice, I took up only the latter. I still sometimes serve clients donuts, croissants or similar desserts, but I try to prepare fruits, healthy biscuits and nuts more often too, so that there is something healthy on offer for my clients. I wore the combination of the striped dress and the scarf with butterflies many more times, because it was one of my favourite combinations and I didn't feel like I was making an unforgivable fashion mistake.

> *Remember: Beech is an intolerant person who criticises sharply and 'without mincing their words' when they wish to point out to others their flaws, mistakes and lapses. By applying this flower remedy, we develop tolerance towards others and acceptance of other people's choices, without the need for criticism.*

CENTAURY

Erythraea centaurium[12]

Dr. Bach's final description of the flower remedy: 'Kind, quiet, gentle people who are over-anxious to serve others. They overtax their strength in their endeavours. Their wish so grows upon them that they become more servants than willing helpers. Their good nature leads them to do more than their own share of work, and in so doing they may neglect their own particular mission in life.'

Description from *The Story of the Travellers* (1934): Indication: '... meek little Centaury so wanted to lighten the burden that he was ready to carry everybody's baggage. Unfortunately for little Centaury, he generally carried the burden of those most able to bear their own because they called

---

[12]   Modern name: *Centaurium umbellatum.*

the loudest.' Positive outcome: '... Centaury ever seeks the weakest who find their burden heavy.'

Group of remedies: for those over-sensitive to influences and ideas

Key words for recognising the remedy: Cinderella, a victim of exploitation, harassment and disrespect

Common expressions: 'It is rude to refuse', 'I have to do it', 'I have to help them', 'I cannot say "no"', 'How can I refuse?'

Personality type: people who are subordinate to others, listen to other people's orders no questions asked, fulfil the wishes of others, while putting themselves in second or last place. They don't know how to fight for themselves or say 'no'. Others take advantage of them and take their kindness and help for granted. A Centaury person allows themselves to be dominated and does not stand up for or defend themselves. When in the company of a dominant person (e.g. Vine), the Centaury person falls silent, bows their head, looks to the floor, obediently does what is required of them.

Examples of situations where we might consider this remedy: in his works Dr. Bach often talks about the relationship between parents and children. Thus he cites several examples in which a person neglects herself/himself, their needs and their life path because they are not able to fight for themselves and say 'no'. These are the examples:

- a person who cares for a sick parent and neglects their partner, their needs or their life path

- a child on whom parents impose the choice of partner, school, college, career, which is different from the child's wishes

- a person who neglects his/her hobbies or life mission because their partner or another person is holding them back (you might also consider Walnut here)

- a person who is abused or harassed by a partner, a parent or another person, if the person cannot stand up for herself and say 'no'

- a person who is always available to help others when they need it, even when they cannot or do not want to help, because they are not able to just say 'no'

Examples of people who might need this flower remedy: a person being abused by a family member or partner, a person being bullied and exploited by their boss – if they cannot say 'no' and stand up for themselves.

Note: flower remedy type that regularly 'plays a role' with Centaury is the Vine type of person.

A Vine person issues orders and Centaury executes them without discussion. Vine bullies, while Centaury is bullied. But it is important to know that one type does not exclude the existence of another type in the same person. In other words, just because you have noticed that a person needs Centaury does not mean that Vine cannot be placed in their bottle, or that the person cannot be in a Vine state. Often a person will be a victim (Centaury) at work and a dictator (Vine) at home, or vice versa. So it is possible for your bottle to contain both types of flower remedies. Likewise, if a person is a Centaury type, she may not be able to confront either the Chicory manipulator, or the Beech person who criticises her, or the Heather person who bothers her with his stories.

Positive outcome of the application of this flower remedy: the person will finally stand up for themselves, say 'no', 'put their foot down', fight for themselves, finally think about themselves and their own needs

'The Story of Centaury Itself', by Dr. Bach (1933)

'I am weak, yes, I know I am weak, but why? Because I have learnt to hate strength and power and dominion, and if I do err a little on the weakness side, forgive me, because it is only a reaction to the hatred of hurting others, and I shall soon learn to understand how to find the balance when I neither hurt nor am hurting. But just for the moment I would rather that I suffered than that I caused one moment's pain to my brother.

So be very patient with your little Centaury, she is weak, I know, but it is a weakness on the right side, and I shall soon grow bigger and stronger and more beautiful until you will all admire me because of the strength I shall bring to you.'

Examples from practice

I had a client whose main problem was work overload. She was in a position that required attending a lot of meetings, working on projects and travelling. Her daughter was still young and she felt that she did not devote enough time to her because of work. The boss often gave her additional tasks when her colleagues were on sick leave, so then she would take over their jobs, stay longer at work; but she never rebelled, even though she was completely exhausted from such a pace and workload. I recommended to put Centaury in her mix, along with Olive for fatigue and exhaustion. At the next consultation, the client told me that the very next day after she had started taking the flower remedies, she went to her boss and expressed her dissatisfaction with being constantly given the assignments of other employees. She said she spoke with such power, uttered such sentences, that she wondered who was saying them and at the same time was in awe at her own strength. For the first time, she stood up for herself and expressed the things that bothered her. She was even afraid that her boss would fire her – that is how determined and direct was she in her outburst. But the boss apologised to her, said she understood her and relieved her of some tasks. This is an example of how we can get into a situation where others take advantage of us and overwhelm us with tasks, if we do not have the strength to fight for ourselves and say openly that we do not have time to do something.

I have had many more such cases in my practice. Most often a person, after taking Centaury flower remedy, can finally say what they think to the person who is harassing, restricting or disrespecting them. For example, one client finally told her employers that she wanted her overtime to be paid. Another client told her husband everything that bothered her in their relationship. I even had a client who decided to move out with his family into a rented apartment because he could no longer bear the interference in their lives of the parents with whom they had lived until then in a shared house. Each of them described the reaction to the Centaury flower remedy in the same way – they got strength they had not had before and they were amazed at themselves, wondering who was speaking in their stead and where their words were coming from.

Remember: Centaury is a tiny flower that gives us tremendous personal strength. It reminds us of the power we already possess but are not aware of. With this remedy, the inferior ones become superior and the weak ones become strong.

CERATO

Ceratostigma willmottiana[13]

Interesting fact: This flower remedy originally grew in Tibet and Dr. Bach found it in the garden of a neighbouring house, which belonged to people who had brought the plant home from a trip to that country.

Dr. Bach's final description of the flower remedy: 'Those who have not sufficient confidence in themselves to make their own decisions. They constantly seek advice from others, and are often misguided.'

Description from *The Story of the Travellers* (1934): Indication: 'Cerato had not much confidence in his judgement and wanted to try every path to be sure they were not wrong …' Positive outcome: 'Cerato knows so well the little paths that lead to nowhere …'

Group of remedies: for uncertainty

Key words for recognising the remedy: distrust in one's own decision-making ability, hesitation after a decision has been made, distrust in one's own intuition

---

[13] The exact name of this plant is *Ceratostigma willmottianum*. The Greek suffix of the word, *-ma*, is not actually of the feminine gender, but The Bach Centre kept *willmottiana* because this name is often used in books on flower essences.

Common expressions: 'I don't know what to choose'; 'What do you think?', 'Which one do you like better?'

Personality type: the person is not sure about their decisions. Indecisive person. They tend to ask for help or advice when choosing and when making a decision, even when it comes to an everyday decision like buying shoes or ordering a meal at a restaurant. They doubt their choice even after having made the decision. These people are at risk of heeding the other person's advice and making a decision based on what the other person has said, not on their inner feeling of what is best for them. A person does not have enough confidence in their intuition. You may notice insecurity in the person's facial expression as well as posture, along with asking for help when making a decision.

Examples of situations where we might consider this remedy: each decision-making action, if the person doesn't trust the decision they have made.

Examples of people who might need this flower remedy: therapists and physicians who need to make a quick and responsible decision about the best therapy for a person and need more confidence in their own decisions.

Positive outcome of the application of this flower remedy: strengthening of one's intuition and developing the ability to make decisions independently.

Note: in the literature you will often read that Cerato or Scleranthus choose between two options, while Wild Oat is the flower remedy for decisions where there are multiple options to choose from. But my experience in practice has shown that all three types of flower remedies can include more than two choices.

So here I want to highlight the difference between these three types of flower remedies intended for decision making, and describe the essential elements for differentiating flower remedies.

CERATO: a decision in case of two or more options, where a person seeks the advice and assistance of other persons when making a decision, and where at some level a decision has been made, but isn't trusted.

SCLERANTHUS: a decision in case of two or more options, where a person does not ask anyone for advice, but tries to find a solution on their own and make a decision, and can't decide.

WILD OAT: a major life decision or choice of life path, when a person is at a turning point in life and a decision has to be made, choosing between two or more options. Wild Oat is about the fundamental path in life we take. Wild Oat lacks a sense of direction and is searching for that.

Examples from practice

One of my clients, who is a Cerato type, always asks for advice, even when it comes to the most trivial decision, and 'suffers' the most in a restaurant when she has to choose a dish. Namely, there is a large selection of dishes and desserts on the menu, so she will often ask everyone at the table what each one of them will order, thus trying to make a decision regarding her own dish. This example shows that

Cerato does not always have to have only two options, but can be sceptical about whether to order pizza, pasta or a salad at a restaurant, which certainly encompasses more than two options. However, the indication for applying Cerato flower remedy is that <u>she asks others to help her with her decision</u>. It often happens that she orders a dish according to what others have recommended to her, but in the end regrets that she did not order something else. Then she either calls the waiter to change her choice or wants to try other dishes, which she did not order. And that is an indication for Cerato flower remedy: people often doubting their decision after the decision has been made.

The same client, on her wedding day, changed her mind at the last minute, changed her shoes and pantyhose right before the wedding, and surprised her hairdresser by deciding to cut her long hair short on the wedding day. Until the last moment, she was asking everyone what to choose and wear from several prepared combinations, and the hairdresser tried several possible hairstyles before the bride made her final decision. It wasn't until she took the flower remedies I recommended to her that she realised exactly what she wanted and made the decisions that were right for her.

Remember: Cerato asks others for help while making a decision and is therefore at risk of making the wrong decision because others will suggest or impose on them not what is best for them or what they would otherwise choose for themselves. This flower remedy helps us trust our intuition and gives us insights that make us realise what is best for us and what we really want.

CHERRY PLUM

Prunus cerasifera

Dr. Bach's final description of the flower remedy: 'Fear of the mind being over-strained, of reason giving way, of doing fearful and dreaded things, not wished and known wrong, yet there comes the thought and impulse to do them.'

Dr. Bach's lecture on this flower remedy: 'The fourth kind of fear is that when there is a dread of the mind being over-worked, and the fear that it cannot stand the strain. When impulses come upon us to do things we should not in the ordinary way think about or for one moment consider. The Remedy for this comes from the CHERRY PLUM, which grows in the hedge-rows around this district. This drives away all the wrong ideas and gives the sufferer mental strength and confidence.'

Group of remedies: for fear

Key words for recognising the remedy: fear of insanity, insanity, loss of control, uncontrolled urge

Common expressions: 'This stress will drive me crazy', 'I could strangle him', 'I feel like hitting him', 'I would like to hit her', 'Everything drives me crazy.'

State of mind: this flower remedy does not represent a personality type, but rather the state of mind that one is in. It is a state of losing control over one's emotions and reactions in moments of excessive pressure and stress.

Note: Loss of control due to stress is a condition that sometimes has the effect of being 'contagious'.

For example, a man comes home from work angry and yells uncontrollably at his wife. The wife, who was in a good mood up until then, enters the child's room and starts yelling at the child uncontrollably, because the child has not yet cleaned their room or done their homework. The child, who until recently had been calmly playing in the room, goes to his younger brother's room and deliberately pushes his brother, who falls to the floor. The boy, angry because his brother had hit him, kicks the dog. From this example, we see that this uncontrolled stress can be 'transmitted' from person to person.

Examples of situations where we might consider this remedy: any situation when our mind is being over-strained, or we fear our reason is giving way, and when we have an impulse to do uncontrollable things.

Examples of people who might need this flower remedy: a parent with many children, children who have tantrums, partners in an argument, any person who has the thought or impulse to do some terrible or crazy things.

Positive outcome of the application of this flower remedy: the person will be able to control their reactions to stress, curb their behaviour and instincts, and act calmly in moments of great pressure or stress. A person gains mental strength and self-control. The thought or urge to do something horrible or scary disappears.

Examples from practice

I usually use this flower remedy in my practice with people who suffer from panic attacks. They very often describe their condition by telling me that they are afraid they will go crazy. They have a feeling that they have no control over their condition and because of that they think they are on the verge of madness. This flower remedy brings them into balance and helps them cope with stress without thinking about some craziness or committing some uncontrolled actions.

I have had on several occasions in consultations parents who discipline their children by pulling their ears or by hitting them, which they said were normal educational measures. In these cases, I recommended Cherry Plum flower remedy, which helps parents maintain self-control. If parents are out of control, this could be Cherry Plum, but if these things are done in a controlled and spiteful way, it is more likely that you would need Holly in this situation.

But there are other indications for the use of this flower remedy. I once had a client who turned to me for help because she had marital problems and was considering filing for divorce. When she talked about her husband, she described very vividly the situations in which she got angry with him and said that she would simply enjoy digging her nails into his back and peeling the skin off his back with her fingernails. Since this flower remedy helps with the <u>thought</u> or <u>impulse</u> to do something crazy and reckless, I recommended Cherry Plum flower remedy to her. But I also added Holly to her combination, as there could be a note of Holly there too: if there is a desire to hurt and take revenge, or spitefulness. After a short time, she smoothed the relationship with her husband and to this day they have remained together in a happy marriage.

Remember: a person in the Cherry Plum state has an idea or an instinct to do something uncontrollably, or even really lose self-control and do something bad in a state of 'madness'. This flower remedy gives us peace of mind in situations of great stress and pressure.

CHESTNUT BUD

Aesculus hippocastanum

Interesting fact: For this flower remedy, buds are collected from the white chestnut tree, just before they turn into flowers.

Dr. Bach's final description of the flower remedy: 'For those who do not take full advantage of observation and experience, and who take a longer time than others to learn the lessons of daily life. Whereas one experience would be enough for some, such people find it necessary to have more, sometimes several, before the lesson is learnt. Therefore, to their regret, they find themselves having to make the same error on different occasions when once would have been enough, or observation of others could have spared them even that one fault.'

Group of remedies: for insufficient interest in present circumstances

Key words for recognising the remedy: repeating the same mistakes over and over again, inability to learn a lesson

Common expressions: 'I don't know why I do this, but I just can't help myself', 'I always make the same mistake', 'I am always late', 'It keeps happening to me and I cannot learn a lesson.'

State of mind: a person who smokes, drinks, overeats, forgets things, is late for work, etc., despite realising it doesn't work out well for him/her, is still doing it, e.g. somebody who is allergic to alcohol but still drinks could benefit from using Chestnut Bud

Examples of situations where we might consider this remedy: the need to master a lesson, such as stopping a child from using diapers or quitting smoking.

Examples of people who might need this flower remedy:

- a person who is always late
- a person who always breaks her/his diet
- a person who always chooses a partner who is not suitable for her/him
- a child being weaned off diapers and not able to learn the lesson
- a person who is always in debt
- an addict who always returns to his vice (cigarettes, gambling, etc.) even though he is aware that it is not good for him
- a person who knows that they will feel nauseous after eating pepperoni or some spicy food, but still eats it every time and later suffers from nausea
- a child who often forgets to bring notebooks to school or forgets to do their homework
- a person who often parks improperly and receives fines

Positive outcome of the application of this flower remedy: the person masters the lesson faster and easier, without suffering the negative consequences of the mistakes they constantly repeat. A person becomes aware of what is good for them and what is wrong, and does what is right for them in the future.

Examples from practice

On one occasion, a client came to me for a consultation and admitted that he was doing a lot of things that he deemed wrong. He would often stay out with friends until the early hours of the morning, over-consume alcohol, smoke and maintain relationships with several women at the same time. He just could not resist it all and even though he knew it was all bad for him, he was still doing all those things and could not stop. After just one bottle of Chestnut Bud, my client came back for the next consultation in amazement. He could not believe how quickly and effectively Bach flower remedies worked. He stopped smoking and drinking alcohol, and chose to continue a relationship with only one lady, whom he knew was good for him, and he was now ready to dedicate himself only to her and treat her well. As he said then, carbonated drinks and coffee remained his only vice. Just one bottle was enough to abandon everything he did wrong. But I must say that he was ready for such a change, because that was exactly the reason why he came for consultations. Even today, after many years, he calls occasionally just to inform me that he is fine and that he is now happily married.

I also have a funny example from my practice, which I want to share with you here.

On one occasion, a client came to me for a consultation because his wife had urged him to. Namely, she wanted him to stop smoking, because she was worried about his health. The gentleman had suffered a heart attack not long before our meeting, from which he had recovered well, but continued to smoke, which his wife considered a great danger to his health. So he came for help to quit smoking. For that purpose, I prepared his personal bottle of Bach flower remedies. After just two days of applying the flower remedies, he called me in amazement, in awe at the power of these flower remedies. And he asked me, 'What magic potion did you give me?' And he said he no longer craved cigarettes, he was not nervous at all and he no longer smoked, after many years of addiction. I explained to him that there was no magic, it was only the normal effect of Bach flower remedies on a person who independently and readily makes the decision to quit smoking.

But after a month, I met that client by chance and saw him with a cigarette in his hand. He was a little embarrassed at first, and it even seemed to me that he would rather hide the cigarette if he could, but it was too late, because I had already seen him. And he started explaining: 'You know, those flower remedies of yours are really magical. Whenever I took them, I could not smoke. I just hated cigarettes and had to put them out. I had a balcony full of cigarettes that were just lit and immediately extinguished. But then one day I found a solution. When I did not take the flower remedies, I did not hate cigarettes – so I could smoke!'

I laughed heartily at this explanation! Well, this is an example of a person who was not ready to quit smoking after all, but had been visibly forced or blackmailed to quit.

That is why I often tell my clients, who have the idea to pour these flower remedies into the coffee or tea of their partners in order to change them, that the flower remedies do not work that way. We cannot force others to change; they must be ready to change. That is why I always say it is not ethical to force someone to use flower remedies, nor to give them flower remedies without their knowledge. If you are bothered by certain traits or habits in your partner, work on yourself first. When your partner sees how well the flower remedies work and how much you change for the better, they will want to try them for themselves. Until then, refrain from manipulation, as this is contrary to the purpose and operation of this system!

Remember: Chestnut Bud flower remedy works only when a person has made the decision to stop doing those things that are bad for them. This flower remedy teaches us not to repeat the same mistakes all the time and shows us the path of proper functioning and living.

CHICORY

Cichorium intybus

Dr. Bach's description of the flower: 'beautiful blue Chicory of the cornfields'

Dr. Bach's final description of the flower remedy: 'Those who are very mindful of the needs of others; they tend to be over-full of care for children, relatives, friends, always finding something that should be put right. They are continually correcting what they consider wrong, and enjoy doing so. They desire that those for whom they care should be near them.'

Description from *The Story of the Travellers* (1934): Indication: 'Chicory had no concern about the end of the journey but was full of solicitude as to whether his fellows were footsore or tired or had enough to eat.' Positive outcome: 'Chicory, always waiting to lend a hand, but only when asked, and then so quietly.'

Group of remedies: for over-care for welfare of others

Key words for recognising the remedy: manipulator, obsessive worrying when a loved one is not near, possessive love

Common expressions: 'I cannot live without you', 'I cannot be without you', 'just stay close to me', 'I know best what is good for you.'

Personality type: manipulator. They stop at nothing to achieve their goal, so that the people they love are under their supervision and control. They use manipulation to get their own way.

Examples of situations where we might consider this remedy: separation from loved ones, when the person cannot bear being apart from their beloved person. For example:

- a parent leaves a baby in the care of another person for the first time
- a child starts going to kindergarten
- a child starts school
- the partner goes on a trip or to their leisure activity or hobby
- the grown-up child leaves home to live independently
- the child goes to study in another city or another country

Examples of people who might need this flower remedy: a parent who is overly anxious about their child/children due to an excessive possessiveness and attachment to them; a husband or wife who possessively supervises their spouse.

Positive outcome of the application of this flower remedy: the person realises that the other person needs to be given trust and freedom. A person learns to be separated from their loved ones.

Differences between Chicory and Beech – correcting what they think is wrong:

The Chicory parent will do the homework instead of their child because they think it helps the child do their best, and does not realise that they are blocking the child's development. The Beech parent will review the child's homework and, without any understanding or tact, criticise the child's work.

Chicory parent will say, 'Let Mummy (Daddy) do it for you.'

Beech parent will say, 'God, how come you don't know that? Alas, this is so stupid or wrong!'

The difference between Chicory and Red Chestnut – concern for the welfare of their loved ones:

A Chicory parent thinks the child cannot go to the store alone because they are going to get lost, even though the child is already ten years old and all their peers are already going alone to school, to the store, and so on, if the cause of this anxiety is excessive possessiveness or excessive attachment to a child. Therefore, here we don't see real fear for the welfare of a child, but possibly manipulation.

The Red Chestnut parent will be concerned about the child if the store is far away or if it is too late for the child to go alone to the store, but in other situations allows the child to leave the house alone.

Chicory parent thinks the child cannot cope without them and is safest if he/she is always with the parent. With Chicory there is an issue of exaggerated attachment between parent and a child, while Red Chestnut is a remedy from a group of remedies for fear, and shows a genuine fear.

Stefan Ball explains the difference between the two with the following examples:[14]

---

[14]   Example from e-mail correspondence with Stefan Ball, regarding the differences between these two remedies.

- 'The difference between Chicory and Red Chestnut is fear. Red Chestnut is anxious that something will happen to a loved one – it's a genuine anxiety – whether or not there is any reason to be afraid. Chicory might say he/she is anxious and only wants to keep the loved one safe, but it's not really fear at all, but a need for affection that leads the Chicory to use manipulation (including claims that 'it's not safe' or 'I am afraid something will happen to you') to keep the loved one close and dependent.'

- '…the Chicory "fear" is assumed, not genuine, and certainly not altruistic as the Red Chestnut fear is.'

The difference between Chicory and Heather – they want people close to them:

Chicory wants the <u>people they love</u> to be with them. They do not tolerate separation from their loved ones. They do not need the company of any person, just for the sake of society, but seek the company of those they love the most. The goal is not to avoid loneliness, but to keep their loved ones under their protection.

A Heather person wants to be close to people (<u>anyone, not necessarily loved ones</u>) because they cannot stand being alone. A Heather will invite a neighbour over for coffee or go to the park to talk to strangers, just to avoid loneliness. The goal is to gain attention and be in the company of any person, just to have someone to talk to and to avoid loneliness.

Examples from practice

I usually give this flower remedy when a child starts going to kindergarten and the mother returns to her job after maternity leave. Then the mother says that she, too, will find it difficult to bear that first separation. In that situation, I recommend Chicory for both mother and baby. Sometimes mothers even shed tears when they tell me that they will be separated from their child. Chicory helps very well in such cases.

Also, I had a few cases where the child was still sleeping with mum in bed while dad spent the night on the sofa, even though the child was about to start going to school and some were even schoolchildren. Progress was made in those cases where the flower remedy was taken by both mother and child. When the mother was not open and not taking the flower remedies herself, the problem would last longer and I would be told at the next consultation that the child was still asking to sleep in bed with the mother or both parents. This is a situation in which one or both parents were not ready to separate. Then, in most cases, it is necessary to repeat taking the personal mix several times.

But I also had a case of a client who came to me because of anxiety. The lady was retired and lived with her husband in Croatia. The son, on the other hand, lived with his wife and children in Germany. The lady was very sad that her son was not around. She told me that she called her son every day and asked him to return to Croatia because she was ill and needed help. She asked him to come back, which he refused. As he rejected her idea, she suffered from repeated anxiety attacks and made frequent visits to the doctor. That story clearly pointed to the need for Chicory flower remedy, because the Chicory person is willing to both manipulate and get sick, or even pretend to be sick, in order to fulfil their goals, and that is primarily to keep their loved ones together.

The client came to me for consultations only twice, after which she called me from Germany. Namely, the flower remedies did their job – she managed to find a solution to her problems. She said her condition had improved and that she was doing fine. But the solution to her problems was actually her decision to move to Germany with her son. In this story, we do not know how the son and daughter-in-law liked the idea of the mother moving in with them and their family, or how her husband reacted to the decision.

In my opinion, it would have been better if she had taken this flower remedy for a while, because in the end she did not balance her condition entirely. But her story is a perfect example of the lengths to which a Chicory person is willing to go to be close to their loved ones.

Remember: A Chicory person cares too much for her loved ones and wants them to be close to her, under her protection. They sometimes exaggerate in this desire, using manipulations when necessary. This flower remedy will loosen the need for supervision, control and manipulation, and teach us lessons on how to give unconditional love, freedom and trust to those we love.

CLEMATIS
Clematis vitalba

Dr. Bach's description of the flower: 'That beautiful plant which adorns our hedges where there is chalk, the Clematis, better known as Traveller's Joy, and whose feathery seeds are, always longing to be blown away and start again, will help you so much to come back and face life and find your work, and bring you joy.'

Dr. Bach's final description of the flower remedy: 'Those who are dreamy, drowsy, not fully awake, no great interest in life. Quiet people, not really happy in their present circumstances, living more in the future than in the present; living in hopes of happier times, when their ideals may come true. In illness some make little or no effort to get well, and in certain cases may even look forward to death, in the hope of better times; or maybe, meeting again some beloved one whom they have lost.'

Group of remedies: for insufficient interest in present circumstances

Key words for recognising the remedy: daydreaming, escape from reality, lack of concentration, head in the clouds, in the world of imagination, dreaming about the future

Common expressions: 'my thoughts wander', 'as if I were in some world of my own', 'as if I lived in the clouds'.

Personality type: an artist, a dreamer. A person does not hear what is being said, as if wandering into the world of imagination, flinching when we ask if he hears what we are telling him.

Examples of situations where we might consider this remedy: poor concentration in school, low concentration on work, when driving a car, doing homework or exams – if the person is in a daydreaming mood.

Examples of people who might need this flower remedy:

- a child whose thoughts wander while learning

- a person who 'zones out' and does not hear what is happening around them because they are playing a game, watching a movie or a game on TV, reading a book, etc.

- a person who has lost a loved one and imagines how they will meet again on the 'other side'

Positive outcome of the application of this flower remedy: the person is present in the now, does not wander into a world of their own, hears what is being said to them.

The difference between Clematis and White Chestnut – lack of concentration:

The White Chestnut person has no concentration because they are disturbed by their own thoughts, which are tormenting them.

Clematis has no concentration because they wander into the world of imagination, which is more interesting than the present they are in.

White Chestnut helps with unwanted and <u>negative</u> thoughts that haunt the mind, while Clematis helps those who are daydreaming about the future and the <u>beautiful</u> things a person fantasises about.

The difference between Clematis and Honeysuckle:

Clematis thinks about the <u>future</u>, which is more beautiful and happier than the present.

Honeysuckle thinks of the <u>past</u>, which was better and happier than the present.

Both people are not present in the now, but live in their thoughts, which can cause the person problems too, because they do not complete a homework assignment, do not complete a report or job project, etc.

'The Story of Clematis Itself', by Dr. Bach (1933)

'And do you wonder that I want to go away? You see, I have fixed my thoughts on earthly things, on earthly people, and if they go I so want to follow them. I just want to fly away and be where they are. Can you blame me? My dreams, my ideal, my romance. Why should I not be with all these things, and what can you offer me that is better? Nothing that I can see. You only offer me cold materialism, life on the earth with all its hardships and sorrows, and there far away is my dream, my ideal. Do you blame me if I follow it?

And Clematis came along and said, "Are your ideals God's ideals? Are you sure that you are serving Him Who made you, Who created you, Who gave you your life, or are you listening just to some other human being who is trying to claim you, and so you are forgetting that you are a son of God with all His Divinity within your soul, and instead of this glorious reality you are being lured away by just some other human being.

I know how we long to fly away to more wonderful realms, but, brothers of the human world, let us first fulfil our duty and even not our duty but our joy, and may you adorn the places where you live and strive to make them beautiful as I endeavour to make the hedges glorious, so that they have called me the 'Travellers' Joy'".'[15]

Examples from practice

One interesting example from my practice was the case of a boy suffering from bronchitis. His mother brought him for a consultation and told me that the boy had recently experienced trauma. Namely, he was very emotionally attached to his grandfather, who had passed away. As the boy was only seven years old, I asked him to tell me a story that was interesting to him, so that I could understand him better and establish communication with him. In a very talkative manner, the boy told me the story of a bird that fell out of its nest and was gone, and the other bird that remained in

---

[15] Travellers' Joy is a country name for the plant *Clematis vitalba*.

the nest is supposed to look for it and go after it. In this story, the metaphor was strong and clear, and it coincided with what the mother had previously told me. The boy was constantly asking his parents if he could visit or go to search for his grandfather, who he missed dearly. I pointed out to the mother the importance of the Clematis flower remedy, because the indication for this flower remedy was strong and identical to the description given by Dr. Bach in his book, meaning that a person looks forward to meeting a dear one who has passed away and is now in the other world. After several consecutive bottles of Clematis flower remedy, the boy became happier and was not so much bothered by sadness.

On the other hand, this is the flower remedy I often use in my practice for children who have difficulty concentrating at school as they are daydreaming during classes, forget what they had for homework, and similar ailments typical of this state of lack of focus.

My daughter Eva is a true example of the Clematis type. From an early age we saw that she would be an artist. She always liked fantasies, drawing, creative games or anything that led her to the beautiful world of her imagination. There were situations when, for example, she would sing while writing homework, or she would write homework and occasionally zone out and look out of the window. Luckily, her teachers mostly had an understanding for her. As she was exactly the Clematis type, it was not easy to balance everything, and I needed a lot of bottles of Clematis to get to a stage where she had a clear focus in school and in learning. But, one day, a turnaround occurred. She became maximally concentrated on learning. She started getting excellent grades, even in the subjects she did not like before, like physics and maths.

Suddenly, it was from these subjects that she began to get the best grades. We predicted she would become an artist, and so she did. She chose to become a professional make-up artist and enrolled in a school for beauticians. Although she is still an artistic type, today she can absolutely maintain focus and concentration in everything she does.

Clematis therefore strengthens concentration and focus in those people who dream and fantasise about a better world in the future.

But here it is necessary to recall another useful application of Clematis flower remedy. Always remember the special application of Clematis flower remedy, and that is a situation in which a person feels dizzy or faints.

On one occasion, I had the opportunity to try this in front of the whole group at the Bach Level 1 seminar. One of the participants felt very dizzy, so I immediately gave her Clematis flower remedy. In a few moments, she was much better and she was no longer dizzy. We later joked that it was just a show for all of us to see how quickly Bach flower remedies work.

I have also given Clematis flower remedy to people who would feel dizzy from the heat.

It might be worth emphasising that in both these cases the remedy was used for the feeling of dizziness, and the feeling of drifting away and losing contact with reality. You should not make a connection between any attack of dizziness and Clematis, as Bach flower remedies are helping with the symptoms of the mind, and not physical diseases and symptoms.

Of course, I am reminding you again that the remedies are not a substitute for emergency medical care!

Remember: Clematis is a flower remedy for dreamers, for those fleeing to the world of imagination and a more beautiful and happier future. This flower remedy brings us back to the present moment and provides us with the focus needed to perform necessary tasks and errands in the present.

CRAB APPLE
Pyrus malus[16]

Dr. Bach's final description of the flower remedy: 'This is the remedy of cleansing. For those who feel as if they had something not quite clean about themselves. Often it is something of apparently little importance: in others there may be more serious disease which is almost disregarded compared to the one thing on which they concentrate. In both types they are anxious to be free from the one particular thing which is greatest in their minds and which seems so essential to them that it should be cured. They become despondent if treatment fails. Being a cleanser, this remedy purifies wounds if the patient has reason to believe that some poison has entered which must be drawn out.'

Group of remedies: for despondency or despair

Key words for recognising the remedy: cleaning, disgust, dissatisfaction with appearance

Common expressions: 'Disgusting!', 'I hate it', 'eww', 'I'm ugly', 'I'm fat', 'I have a big nose', 'I have lop ears.'

Personality type: a Crab Apple person will always express disgust. Such a person constantly washes their hands, cleans

---

[16]   Modern name: *Malus sylvestris.*

the house, wipes the dust, disinfects everything around them, etc. Similarly, it may be that the person does not like some part of his/her body or does not consider themselves beautiful, and thus acts constantly, not just in a particular situation. This is, for example, a person who is obese, who has a big nose, or generally does not consider themselves beautiful. Such people usually do not like to be photographed and do not accept compliments. It is also possible for such people to undergo cosmetic surgery or develop bulimia or anorexia, the reason being dissatisfaction with their own appearance.

Examples of situations where we might consider this remedy:

- a person in the family has a cold, virus or some infectious disease, and a household member who falls into the Crab Apple state then has a fear of infection, washes their hands constantly, avoids the person who sneezes, coughs, wipes their nose, etc.

- a person is invited to a wedding and needs to dress up and put on a formal dress, and they think they are fat, so that's what they focus all their attention on and feel fat

- a person has a pimple on their face and all day their focus is on whether someone will notice it, and they are just thinking about how to cover it up

- a person travels to a foreign country where hygiene is less developed and everything disgusts them

- the person uses a public loo and feels that everything around them is dirty

- the person goes to the doctor, where sick people are sitting in the waiting room, coughing and wiping their noses, and then they feel disgusted and think they will get infected

- the person has a viral or bacterial infection and feels dirty because of it
- the person is taking an antibiotic or a medicine and has a feeling that the medicine is harming them and that toxins are circulating in their body; the same goes for vaccines and other therapies that this person considers poison
- the person has a skin disease or a sexually transmitted disease and feels contaminated

Examples of people who might need this flower remedy: people who are dissatisfied with their appearance and are considering cosmetic surgery or have already undergone cosmetic procedures. People who have anorexia or bulimia, where the cause is dissatisfaction with their appearance. People who have acne, a skin disease or some infectious disease like sexually transmitted diseases, AIDS, etc., and as a result they feel dirty and contaminated.

Positive outcome of the application of this flower remedy: the person will become more satisfied with their appearance and will no longer think that everyone is 'staring' at them or that everyone sees that flaw from afar. The person will have more self-confidence regarding their appearance, will start to dress up, go out, and will react positively to compliments, smile and say 'thank you'. The person will no longer be overly afraid of infections, nor will everything around them be a source of disgust.

The difference between Crab Apple and Larch – lack of self-confidence:

Crab Apple lacks self-confidence regarding their appearance and body.

Larch lacks self-confidence regarding their knowledge, skills and the work they do.

The difference between Crab Apple and Rock Water – need for cleaning and tidiness:

Crab Apple cleans the house to avoid germs.

Rock Water cleans the house as s/he likes order and perfection.

Examples from practice

There are well-known stories about how famous inventor Nikola Tesla had a phobia of bacteria, dirt, infection and microbes. He asked for a clean tablecloth for every meal, and he always wiped every dish and cutlery with a napkin before eating. The napkin was never used twice, not even during one meal. He would refuse to shake hands due to his fear of germs.

Today there are also many people who have the same phobias, and this is exactly what Dr. Bach wrote about – that Bach flower remedies will have the same application in his time, in a hundred years, and always, because people behave in the same way, even though the circumstances in which we live change.

Today some of my clients are terrified of foods that they believe will make them sick – gluten, lactose, soy, nuts, etc. Some avoid many foods, even though they do not harm them personally, but have only read about it. I have often had clients who carry their water bottles and their own food, and eat only in well-tested places, for fear of infection and foods that can harm them. In all such situations, I recommended the Crab Apple remedy. Equally, this remedy has helped greatly in cases with young ladies who were deeply unsatisfied with their looks and suffered from anorexia. During our conversation, they kept repeating how fat they were and how they had to control their food intake to keep from gaining weight, and at the same time it had nothing to do with reality. These were all beautiful and slender girls but, unfortunately, deeply dissatisfied with themselves. In these cases I also recommended Crab Apple.

It is good to take this flower remedy in all situations where a person is overwhelmed by fear of infection, when a person is constantly thinking about it, for example during the flu season, during a visit to a doctor's office or while flying in an airplane.

At the moment, as I am writing these examples, the media is constantly reporting on the Covid-19 virus that keeps spreading. People are in a panic, they move away from other people, and if someone accidentally coughs, everyone around them immediately gets upset, fearing infection. This is one of the most important flower remedies to take at this time if the person is constantly thinking about the virus. Of course, this flower remedy does not provide protection against viruses or bacteria, but it does help a person not to be overwhelmed by thoughts about it and to be able to continue to function normally in all their daily activities.

 Remember: Crab Apple flower remedy gives us satisfaction with our own appearance, frees us from disgust and excessive worry about cleanliness, and prevents our mind from constantly thinking about our physical defects, infections, viruses and bacteria.

ELM

Ulmus campestris[17]

Dr. Bach's final description of the flower remedy: 'Those who are doing good work, are following the calling of their life and who hope to do something of importance, and this often for the benefit of humanity. At times there may be periods of depression when they feel that the task they have undertaken is too difficult, and not within the power of a human being.'

Group of remedies: for despondency or despair

Key words for recognising the remedy: overburdened with obligations

Common expressions: 'I cannot do everything at once', 'the day has only 24 hours', 'I work for three people', 'I would manage to do everything if only I did not sleep.'

Personality type: a person who is otherwise capable and can perform all the tasks entrusted to them, but due to too much work or too little time, they are not able to complete all of the tasks. Because of this, they enter a state of frustration or overload with obligations. Exhaustion, stress, nervousness and haste occur.

Examples of situations where we might consider this remedy: overload with numerous obligations, insomnia due to thinking about their excessive obligations.

Examples of people who might need this flower remedy: this flower remedy is suitable for every person who is overburdened with obligations, for every person who is overworked because after work you also need to cook dinner and

---

[17] Modern name: *Ulmus procera.*

tidy up and run some additional errands; for every person who both studies and works, for every person working two jobs, for every parent who has several children, etc., if they feel over-burdened with responsibilities.

Positive outcome of the application of this flower remedy: after applying this flower remedy, it is not to be expected that the obligations a person has will miraculously disappear. The obligations will still be there, but the person will now know how to prioritise. For those obligations that are less important and can be delegated to someone else, the person will do so or ask for help to solve them. After applying this flower remedy, a person will, for the first time, be able to refuse a task that they know they will not be able to complete. Also, they will regain confidence in themselves, about their ability to handle many overwhelming tasks.

Note: if a person is not able to say 'no', it is necessary to add Centaury to the personal mix.

The difference between Impatiens and Elm – handling work assignments:

Impatiens is eager to get the job done quickly because he/she cannot stand slowness and waiting.

Elm is concerned because there are a lot of other tasks to be finished and he/she is worried about whether they will get everything done.

Elm does not delegate tasks, but tries to complete all tasks on time, because they consider themselves capable of completing them.

Impatiens takes other people's tasks on to themselves because they cannot bear to watch their slowness in carrying out the tasks and think that they can do everything faster and better on their own.

The difference between Elm and Oak – responsibility:

Elm is capable and responsibly performs the tasks assigned to them. But they break down or get sick when overwhelmed with obligations, and when unable to complete them all due to lack of time or overlapping obligations. They give up under the burden of responsibilities and obligations.

Oak is capable and does tasks responsibly because they have a sense of duty and responsibility to other people. Oak fulfils all obligations, even if they do not sleep and even if they collapse from fatigue, because they cannot break the obligation or promise they gave to others. At the cost of their health, they will perform all the tasks and will never give up.

Examples from practice

The Elm flower remedy is one of the most commonly used flower remedies in my practice. I like to explain to clients that this is the result of the hustle and bustle of the age in which we live. It is a novelty brought to us by the fast-food and telecommunications industries. Everything needs to be available and resolved now and immediately. We are all available to everyone on a laptop or mobile phone, so the work is done both at home and while on vacation. For a lot of people, working hours no longer exist, and obligations have multiplied many times over. It is normal for women to be employed and to raise children at the same time, take care of the household and family, and in addition to all that it is necessary to be well groomed, to have hobbies, to find the time for oneself, friends, for reading a book, etc. That is why this flower remedy is needed by many of my clients who are overworked. But, besides Elm, other remedies might be also suitable for this modern and busy lifestyle, depending on the individual. As we all react differently, different people might need different remedies. Elm is one of the common ones, but not exclusive.

I must mention here that in my practice I have also seen a lot of children who are overburdened with obligations. Namely, a lot is expected from today's children and a much greater burden is placed on them than the one we had when we were growing up. For example, children today are taught from an early age that they must enrol in college and must have excellent grades in school, without exception. Children have a lot of extracurricular activities, where they are again expected to excel. In my day, when I was a child, my generation did not have that much pressure. Again, reactions to overload can be different, as children are different, but Elm is certainly one of the remedies to consider. Always ask the person how he/she feels in that situation to discover the right remedies.

Nowadays I also see that parents are overly protective of their children (Chicory), so parents take on the obligation to drive their children to all extracurricular activities, do their homework with them or read their children's reading material, thus causing even greater overload.

Unfortunately, the Elm tree is an endangered species today and is threatened with extinction. 'In recent decades, the elm tree has been attacked by Dutch elm disease (*Ceratostamella ulmi*). Infested trees dry up abruptly. The cause is a fungus, and it is transmitted by bark beetles. In our country [in Croatia, author's note], 30–50% of elms have withered due to this disease.'[18]

It is sad for me to see that the tree whose essence is of great help to so many people today is facing extinction. It is another in a series of alarming conditions that people need to take seriously and I do hope Elm trees will recover from this.

 Remember: Elm helps us when we are overwhelmed with obligations to prioritise, delegate tasks and seek help when we need it, instead of giving up under the burden of obligations.

GENTIAN
Gentiana amarella

Dr. Bach's description of the flower: '… the little Gentian of our hilly pastures will help you to keep your firmness of purpose, and a happier and more hopeful outlook even when the sky is over-cast. It will bring you encouragement at all times, and the understanding that there is no failure when you are doing your utmost, whatever the apparent result.'

Dr. Bach's final description of the flower remedy: 'Those who are easily discouraged. They may be progressing well in illness or in the affairs of their daily life, but any small delay or hindrance to progress causes doubt and soon disheartens them.'

---

[18] 'Elm tree – why is elm a very rare tree today?', https://www.rtl.hr/zivotistil/vrt-i-sobno-bilje/2997561/brijest-drvo-zasto-je-danas-brijest-vrlo-rijetko-drvo/ (accessed 19 January 2020).

Group of remedies: for uncertainty

Key words for recognising the remedy: discouragement after a setback

Common expressions: 'I will surely fail the exam again', 'The same thing as last time will happen again.'

State of mind: a person who is discouraged after an initial failure, takes on other people's negative experiences as their own.

Examples of situations where we might consider this remedy:

- taking an exam after having previously failed it
- a new relationship after the breakup of a previous love affair, or after divorce
- artificial insemination after a failed last attempt
- new pregnancy after a miscarriage or a difficult birth
- a new job after a dismissal or failure at a previous job
- making friends after a friend has let one down
- flying on an airplane after experiencing turbulence during the last flight
- new diet after the last diet failed
- new therapy after the last therapy failed
- a new game or race after a lost match or race

… if a person feels discouraged afterwards.

Examples of people who might need this flower remedy: anyone who is feeling discouraged after a setback or failure.

Positive outcome of the application of this flower remedy: the person will have faith that they will succeed. The person will not automatically predict a negative outcome of the situation. The person will think positively.

Examples from practice

I recently had a case of a client who is an entrepreneur and who was very discouraged because several regular clients had terminated their contractual relationship with the company he ran. He said that it seemed to him that, every time, he actually starts the business year from a scratch, as if he were a beginner in the business world, because he always needs to renegotiate contracts at the beginning of each year. Such a situation burdened him greatly and he felt discouraged. I suggested he took Gentian for a few weeks, after which he felt better and no longer felt the burden of closing contracts with clients.

Another wonderful application of Gentian flower remedy is for people who suffer from cancer or some other condition or disease, and one method of treatment has failed to help them. This flower remedy helps them to stay positive and try with another method of treatment. The same can be applied to people who have problems with high blood pressure and doctors are still trying to prescribe the right medicine or the right dose of medicine to keep their blood pressure stable. Gentian is the flower remedy that gives them the confidence that these negative episodes will not happen again and that the right cure or medicine will be available for them.

After a person takes this flower remedy, they get the feeling: 'this time everything will be fine' and 'now I will succeed'. They simply always have hope and are willing to try again.

Here I still have to tell the story of a wonderful woman, whom I have known practically all my life. I have told her story a hundred times – when it would become all too hard for my clients and they would feel discouraged – and I always said I would put her story in a book one day. And now I am telling this story as a continuation of Dr. Bach's quote with which I began writing about this flower remedy.

This is the story of a woman who remained firm in achieving her goal, a happy and more positive attitude, even when the sky was overcast. This is the story of Jadranka Pongrac, her husband Miroslav and their children. Jadranka is a professional athlete with the highest international success. She also has her own tailoring salon. This story is difficult, but it is also very special. Namely, the most terrible thing in life happened to this married couple. Their only son, Tin, died just before his fifth birthday from the consequences of a brain tumour. I was a student at the time. Jadranka is my sister Silvija's best friend, so I followed these events with great sadness. I must say that after Tin's death, I developed headaches and insomnia from the shock, and felt great sadness for months to follow. I cannot even imagine how Jadranka and Miro must have felt! But while this is a sad story, it has a very inspiring sequel. For a certain period of time, they tried to conceive again. Subsequent pregnancies were unfortunately ectopic. But Jadranka never gave up or lost hope. In fact, all those days after the departure of their little angel Tin, she dedicated herself to sports, her husband, the future. She did not lose hope. Very soon, some three years after the unfortunate event, Jadranka and Miro made the decision to adopt a child. Little 15-month-old David became a new member of their family. Three years later, their family was enlarged with two more adopted boys – Luka and Sandro. The sons always listened to the story of Tin, who in a way made it possible for the three of them to find a happy home and wonderful parents. Today, these boys are adults. Jadranka and Miro having literally enacted the well-known saying: 'When God closes a door, somewhere He opens a window.' They turned their difficult and sad story into an inspiring one that can be an example for many. They transformed their grief into happiness for the three little ones. They discovered their new mission and their new purpose. How many times have I told this story ... And now I have fulfilled what I always said I would do – the story of this family is now written down.

For additional inspiration, here are the original words of Jadranka, which she wrote especially for you readers and for this book of mine:

'My name is Jadranka Pongrac. I was born on August 31, 1968, in Zagreb. I am married, I have a wonderful husband Miroslav and four sons. In 1991, I gave birth to my beautiful boy Tin. At the age of five, on April 4, 1996, he became our angel – a celestial flyer. After I had an ectopic pregnancy (EP) in 1997, in 1999 my husband and I decided to adopt a child. On January 31, 2000, we got David. He was 15 months old then. After a couple of years I had a second EP, and on July 1, 2003, we adopted two more boys. Sandro was six and Luka was four and a half.

With them, our life is full of vivacity. We helped them, but they taught us how to live.

I have been training judo since I was 11 years old. I am a 6th day black belt holder. I am an international judo and kata judge. Judo is part of my life.

I graduated from textile school, as a tailor, and then at the Faculty of Textile Technology as a clothing designer. I have a tailoring salon and I enjoy rummaging through cloths.

I have had several surgeries for tumours, cancers and similar growths that can interfere with physical health, but with love, prayer, and judo, the body and spirit have healed.

I believe in God and the power of prayer. The latter is an integral part of my life and guides me through all life situations. It teaches me to live in all spheres of my life.'

Jadranka Pongrac

At the time, Jadranka did not have Bach flower remedies to help her, but this story shows us what it looks like when a person already has the built-in positive qualities of Gentian flower remedy.

 Remember: Gentian flower remedy helps us to see any new attempt after failure as a new experience, without fear that the unwanted situation will happen again. This flower remedy teaches us to get up after a fall and boldly move on to success and victory!

GORSE

Ulex europaeus

Dr. Bach's final description of the flower remedy: 'Very great hopelessness, they have given up belief that more can be done for them. Under persuasion or to please others they may try different treatments, at the same time assuring those around that there is so little hope of relief.'

Description from *The Story of the Travellers* **(1934):** Indication: 'Gorse lost all hope and said, "I can go no further; you go along, but I shall stay here as I am until death relieves my sufferings."' Positive outcome: 'Gorse in the blackest night tells them of the progress they will make when the sun rises in the morning.'

Group of remedies: for uncertainty

Key words for recognising the remedy: giving up

Common expressions: 'Never again!', 'I don't want to try again!', 'There is no way it is going to work', 'There is no sense in trying', 'It's over!'

State of mind: pessimistic mood, gloomy and negative people

Examples of situations where we might consider Gorse remedy:

- retaking an exam after having previously failed it
- a new relationship after a breakup or divorce
- artificial insemination after an attempt that failed
- new pregnancy after a miscarriage or difficult birth
- new job after dismissal from previous job
- making friends after a friend has let one down
- flying an airplane after experiencing turbulence during the previous flight
- new diet after the last failed diet
- new therapy after the last failed therapy

- a new match or race after a lost match or race

... if a person is hopeless and gives up afterwards.

Examples of people who might need this flower remedy: a person who gives up and has no hope; this might be after a setback, or without even trying for a solution or a cure.

Positive outcome of the application of this flower remedy: the person, after applying this flower remedy, will realise that each new situation is a new experience and that success is possible if they try again. Hope for success revives.

The difference between Gentian and Gorse remedies – discouragement:

Situation	Gentian	Gorse
Discouragement	Has hope	Has no hope
Failing an exam	Thinks they will fail the exam again, but they take the exam	Gives up university studies
Breakup or divorce	Thinks the same thing will happen again in the next relationship or marriage	Decides not to enter into a new relationship or marriage
Failed artificial insemination	Thinks the same thing will happen again, but they will try again	Gives up artificial insemination
New pregnancy after miscarriage or difficult childbirth	Thinks the same thing will happen again, but they will try again	Gives up on pregnancy
New job after dismissal from previous job	Thinks they will get fired again, but still looks for a new job	Gives up looking for a new job
Making friends after a friend let them down	Thinks someone will let them down again, but makes friends and hangs out with friends	Never trusts anyone again and isolates him/herself from others

Flying on a plane after experiencing turbulence during the previous flight	Worries that the same thing will happen again, but flies on a plane	Does not fly on a plane again
New diet after the last diet failed	S/he thinks s/he won't be able to lose weight, but s/he goes on a diet again	Gives up the diet
New therapy after the last therapy failed	Thinks that the next therapy won't help either, but will try it anyway	Does not agree to the new therapy
A new game or race after a lost match or race	Thinks they will lose again, but will do their best and go to the next competition	Gives up further competition
The bank rejected the loan application	Submits the application to another bank, although they think it will be rejected by that bank too	Gives up asking for a loan and does not send the application to any other bank
Reaction to any situation in which she/he experiences failure	Tries again, but doubts their chances of success	Gives up: 'Never again!'

The difference between Gentian, Gorse and Sweet Chestnut flower remedies – giving up:

Gentian has hope, but is afraid they will once again fail.

Gorse has no hope. Gorse has given up and does not want to try again after failing.

Sweet Chestnut has hope, but has come to the point where the suffering and emotional pain are too unbearable and make it impossible to go on.

Sweet Chestnut gives up after trying everything in their power, while Gorse gives up because they think they have no solution and no hope of succeeding.

In case of depression or illness, these three flower remedies react as follows:

- Gentian has hopes of recovery and is trying various therapies and treatment methods, but fears they will not recover.

- Gorse gives in to a negative diagnosis and prognosis, and has no hope that they will recover. They do not seek another opinion, therapy or alternative methods. Even if they agree to a method because others have persuaded them, they have no hope and do not believe in healing.

- Sweet Chestnut has hope, but the emotional pain they experience is unbearable and insufferable, so the person has reached the limits of their endurance. Suffering and agony are too strong and too painful.

Maybe you will understand best the difference between Gentian, Gorse and Sweet Chestnut with the example of a case of artificial insemination …

Gentian has hope and tries again and again, although previous rounds of artificial insemination were not successful. Gentian doubts they can succeed, but tries and hopes.

Gorse gives up after one (or more) attempts at unsuccessful artificial insemination. They believe that there is no hope and there is no chance that artificial insemination would result in pregnancy.

Sweet Chestnut has hope. Although a previous round of artificial insemination has not resulted in pregnancy, Sweet Chestnut is desperately trying all alternative methods that could help her get pregnant, and tries artificial insemination again and again. A Sweet Chestnut person will give up artificial insemination only when the suffering and the emotional pain of disappointment become so unbearable that they can no longer endure them. The Sweet Chestnut person gives up artificial insemination only when they have exhausted all possibilities, and when they believe that one more attempt would destroy them mentally and physically, and they are not ready to go through the suffering and pain of unsuccessful artificial insemination again.

Examples from practice

In my practice and work with people, I have noticed an interesting thing: a person can enter the Gentian or Gorse state based on the failure of others. For example, a child of divorced parents may, based on the experience that his or her parents had when going through divorce, adopt the following belief:

Gentian: *I plan to get married one day, but maybe I'll get a divorce one day too, because it's hard to keep a marriage going.*

Gorse: *I will never get married! Marriage is doomed anyway and it's not worth trying.*

I came to this realisation after witnessing several almost identical cases of women in their forties who never married. They all talked about their traumatic childhood and the divorce of their parents, from which they learned that one should not bond or marry. But they were not happy as a result of this decision, and they felt lonely and unhappy (which was an indication for some other flower remedies too, not only Gorse).

Also, several clients during my practice have told me that they stand firm in their decision not to marry officially with their partner with whom they live, because they have previously gone through the experience of the divorce of their parents. But the resulting emotional state they were in was enough of an indicator to recommend Gorse flower remedy to them.

I would hate to think that this section sounds like I believe that deciding not to get married is somehow 'wrong' and needs treating. If somebody decides not to get married, this alone does not require any remedies at all, as long as the person is happy with this decision. Oprah Winfrey herself has emphasised many times in her interviews that it was her choice not to get married to her partner Stedman, and that they are perfectly happy this way. If someone is happy and in balance, they don't need any remedies at all! But, if a decision not to get married is causing them to be unhappy, if their partner is unhappy, if their relationship is undergoing problems as the other partner wants to get married, or if the person feels anger and resentment towards their ex-wife or ex-husband, and the decision not to get married is making them feel unhappy and unbalanced, then we can decide on the remedies based on the emotions they are experiencing.

I have noticed the same adoption of other people's experiences and beliefs in women who are planning pregnancy. If some of their friends battled a difficult birth, or could not get pregnant, they themselves have accepted other people's experiences as their own, and initially looked at pregnancy and childbirth through the eyes of others. Listening to the stories of others, some women have developed a belief that their childbirth will be difficult, that they will not be able to breastfeed, that they will not be able to conceive, and the like, and they feared failure based solely on other people's experiences. For such negative beliefs, I regularly recommended Gentian. For those women who did not plan to give birth or get pregnant, or breastfeed at all, because they heard stories that it was difficult and painful, through the recommendation of Gorse remedy, these women opened up to the possibility of one day getting pregnant and having a child. But I did not recommend the remedy to reassure them that they had made the wrong decision, but because there were indications that deep down they wanted a child and were not happy with their decision. I repeat, Bach flower remedies are needed only when a person is in a negative state, and those who are happy and satisfied and in a positive state of mind do not need any therapy.

Additional advice: My recommendation to pregnant women and women planning a pregnancy is therefore always: 'Shut your ears when someone is telling you about their (negative) experience of pregnancy, childbirth, breastfeeding.' Also, do not read in advance about diseases and complications. You will read about them only if such a situation really occurs.

I personally took Gorse after I lost twins in my fourth pregnancy. This helped me realise I did want to try again, but was only afraid of another miscarriage (this is also an indication for Mimulus). Sadly, my fifth pregnancy did not turn out well either, so I really did give up. I was not ready to go through yet another painful episode like this. But after a while, I took Gorse again, just to see how the remedy would act. Actually, it did revive my desire to have more children, and I was not scared of another miscarriage. But our efforts to conceive again did not result in pregnancy, and eventually we made peace with the fact it was not meant to be. But I still hold this positive feeling inside me – that pregnancy is nothing to be feared! Gorse did help, and I am happy I took it as it cleared away my fear and trauma from past negative events.

I also applied Gorse flower remedy when I was writing my doctoral thesis, as I stated in the introductory part of this book. When I was almost done writing – I only needed to write about thirty pages more as a conclusion and it would be finished (out of a total of 533 pages) – I no longer had the strength to write. I turned off the computer and told my husband I could not write any more and that I was giving up. I even went to see my mentor and explained to him that I would not submit my thesis on time and that it was possible I would fail to get my doctoral degree. He looked at me in honest astonishment and disbelief, but then he realised that I was on the verge of exhaustion and not joking. He called the office of convocation to check what the last day was for the official submission of papers to the Commission. The lady from the office said that we only have seven days left to hand in the work. I went home, pleased to have expressed my intention of imminent withdrawal. I put together a bottle of Gorse flower remedy and sipped it throughout the day. I rested for an entire five days and did not write a single letter in those days. Then I sat down, typed the last thirty pages of my dissertation in one afternoon, and handed in my doctorate on time. Gorse flower remedy just won't let us give up when we're so close to the goal.

Gorse flower remedy gives us the motivation to persevere, no matter how hopeless the situation may seem to us.

 Remember: Gorse flower remedy gives us back hope for success and provides us with the strength to try again. To endure and persevere, to move on – that is the strength that this flower remedy gives.

HEATHER

Calluna vulgaris

Dr. Bach's final description of the flower remedy: 'Those who are always seeking the companionship of anyone who may be available, as they find it necessary to discuss their own affairs with others, no matter who it may be. They are very unhappy if they have to be alone for any length of time.'

Group of remedies: for loneliness

Key words for recognising the remedy: chatterbox, hypochondriac

Common expressions: 'let me tell you this', 'my', 'myself', and 'I' all the time.

Personality type: a Heather person does not like to be alone and cannot stand loneliness. Such a person will seek the company of anyone who is willing to listen to them. In fact, they are looking for a 'victim' who will listen to their stories – without interrupting them and without talking about themselves. Namely, the Heather person is so self-centred that they do not care about other people's problems. They find their problems to be the greatest and need to talk about them with everyone and at every opportunity. Heather is a person who, when they are alone at home, will call one person at a time, just so they do not feel lonely. Maybe she will invite a neighbour over for coffee or will go over to the neighbour's herself. If one person does not answer the phone, they will call someone else. If they cannot find an interlocutor in any other way, because over time people start to avoid them, then they will go to shops, the pharmacy or the doctor's, where they find new 'victims' who will (have to) listen to their problems and stories. When Heather talks, it is hard to interrupt them. When you manage to say something, Heather will quickly interrupt your story and will start to talk again about themselves and their problems. The Heather person will tell you details about their family, about events at work, about other people they are connected to and their problems, about the details of their illness(es) and all their hardships (you will know exactly what was their blood pressure in the morning, noon and evening), about all the medications they take, about what they eat, etc. The Heather person often talks quickly, talks a lot, and comes closer to you if you try to walk away.

Examples of situations where we might consider this remedy: any condition in which a person is self-centred and wants to talk about themselves and their problems or life events, but are not otherwise Heather type, and only current circumstances lead them to talk about themselves, such as in the following phases or situations, for example:

- the person has learned they have a disease and needs to tell others about it
- a pregnant woman who needs to tell everyone about her pregnancy
- a parent who has had a baby and needs to talk about everything that is happening to the child
- after a trip she or he wants to tell everyone about it
- the loss of a loved one or loss of pregnancy, which they need to talk about to everyone
- change of job, when one feels the need to tell people about the reasons for the change

- breakup and the need to tell about all related details
- new relationship and the need to tell about all related details

Examples of people who might need this flower remedy: people who live alone, people who are seriously ill, pregnant women, people suffering from panic attacks, people who are retired, single people, etc. – if there is a need to talk to others about their problems or situation.

Positive outcome of the application of this flower remedy: a person realises that they are not the centre of the world and that other people have their problems, often bigger than theirs. They can readily listen to other people. They can refrain from talking only about themselves and their problems.

The difference between Heather and Vervain – talkativeness:

Heather talks about themselves and their problems or about life situations they are going through. A Heather person is self-centred and not interested in the problems and stories of others. Their only goal is for someone to listen to them and not to be alone.

Vervain talks about their beliefs, and the things they deeply believe in and practise, which they think other people would find useful too if they adopted and applied them. Vervain talks a lot because they want to convince others that they can help them. Vervain talks a lot because they think it will help their interlocutor.

Examples from practice

It's easy to work with Heather people. Unlike Agrimony, who is the complete opposite, who hides their problems from you and does not want to reveal anything personal about themselves, Heather will tell you everything – both what is important for you to determine the content of their personal mix, as well as what is irrelevant; what interests you and what does not interest you. The only rule with Heather people is to keep track of how long the consultation lasts, so that the next client does not have to wait long. Because Heather can talk for hours.

My experience with Heather is that they are usually well-meaning people, eager for someone to listen to them. There are those who are so kind and charming in their 'Heather' performance, that you can listen to them for days. I have to say that I was obviously lucky because the Heather people in my environment and all my Heather clients were positive, likeable and kind people. Maybe the thing is that I perfectly understand the needs of a Heather person, so I let them tell me everything about themselves, so that they got exactly what they were looking for – a pair of ears that would listen to them.

I also have Heather friends and a few dear Heather people in my life. What is important for a Heather person is that you know that they are not naughty or rude people because they do not ask about your problems or because they do not listen to your stories. They are simply so preoccupied with themselves that they are not aware that you may also need to tell them something.

And remember how I told you at the beginning of the book that I tried every single Bach flower remedy? I tried Heather too – several times! I had my Heather phases during panic attack episodes, during divorce proceedings and after lost pregnancies. And I must tell you it was pretty 'painful' to realise I was in a Heather state - and possibly annoying to others. But, as I have said, these are all states that we all go through in life, and we need to look to all Bach flower remedies as our helpers.

In practice, I often recommended Heather flower remedy to those people who were going through difficult life situations, the kinds of situation where they needed to talk to anyone willing to listen to them: a man whose wife had died, a woman left by her husband and left alone with three children, a woman who found a new love after divorce, a woman who has been ill since childhood and suffers from a multitude of ailments, a woman who is a company director, and has a need to talk about all the details of her business and private problems, and a woman who lives alone. Also, a lot of people who suffer from panic attacks and are considered hypochondriacs have visited my centre, so they were focused on observing their problems all day long, and even the smallest physical symptom would easily upset them. They all felt relief after applying Heather flower remedy.

 Remember: Heather flower remedy helps us find peace and contentment within ourselves, to relax in moments of solitude, to enjoy peace and quiet, to listen to others and to help others. With this flower remedy, 'me, myself and I' fades into the background and we begin to realise that holding a conversation is a two-way street, not one-directional communication.

HOLLY
Ilex aquifolium

Dr. Bach's final description of the flower remedy: 'For those who sometimes are attacked by thoughts of such kind as jealousy, envy, revenge, suspicion. For the different forms of vexation. Within themselves they may suffer much, often when there is no real cause for their unhappiness.'

Group of remedies: for those over-sensitive to influences and ideas

Key words for recognising the remedy: hatred, spitefulness, jealousy, envy, suspiciousness, revenge

Common expressions: 'I hate that person', 'one day I will get my revenge for that', 'I'm glad it happened to them, they deserve it.'

State of mind: a vengeful, envious and suspicious person. The person has hatred and envy in their eyes.

Examples of situations where we might consider this remedy: quarrel, breakup, anger – if the person feels emotions like hatred, spitefulness, jealousy, envy, suspiciousness, revenge, etc.

Examples of people who might need this flower remedy: jealousy and envy among colleagues at work, jealousy and envy of someone else's beauty or success, jealousy and envy among siblings, people who are jealous and suspicious in their love relationship, people who are going through a breakup, spouses who have marital problems, divorced ex-spouses who hurt each other, desire for revenge against a former employer.

Positive outcome of the application of this flower remedy: a person finds love and understanding for other people, is willing to forgive and forget, is willing to offer a second chance to others, and is capable of seeing the situation from another person's perspective.

Note: in my practice, Holly is the remedy that has innumerable times reconciled people who had a quarrel or people facing divorce, and those people have again found love and understanding for each other. Even when only one of them took this flower remedy, it so happened that the other person also began to show more love, as the person who took the flower remedy began to change.

Examples from practice

Here is an example from practice, when I recommended Scleranthus in combination with Holly (for a story, see the example provided for Scleranthus flower remedy). For a clearer indication for Holly flower remedy, the sections that accurately describe the effect of the Holly after just one day of using the remedy are underlined.

'I have been married for a couple of years, during which time I went through a lot of stressful life phases. In all of this, my relationship with my husband suffered, since I felt he did not give me enough support.

I can say that for a couple of years I was torn, pondering upon whether we should part or not [this is an indication for Scleranthus flower remedy, author's note]. The interesting thing was that my love for him was quite intense at first.

I told Ana how I was feeling, my dilemmas, etc. and then a miracle followed. The first day, maybe in the middle of the second day, I loved him so much, that my soul was filled with fire! I cannot explain that feeling in any other way!!!

That is how Bach flower remedies helped me see that I still had emotions for him. If I hadn't tried them, God knows what would have happened to us, and now we and our child are enjoying every minute of expecting our second child.'

I have many more cases like this to tell. Always with the same effect. The person finds the love in his or her heart again.

Holly flower remedy helped both me and my husband during our divorce. We never hurt each other, and we maintained a civilised and friendly relationship even during the separation phase. Holly guarded our love and showed us the way of love again.

> *Remember: Holly flower remedy erases hatred, jealousy, envy and suspicion towards others, and incites love and positive feelings in us towards everyone around us. Holly forgives and allows us to let go of certain things. Holly melts and warms the icy heart. Holly removes the thorns and fences we surround ourselves with.*

HONEYSUCKLE
Lonicera Caprifolium

Dr. Bach's final description of the flower remedy: 'Those who live much in the past, perhaps a time of great happiness, or memories of a lost friend, or ambitions which have not come true. They do not expect further happiness such as they have had.'

Group of remedies: for insufficient interest in present circumstances

Key words for recognising the remedy: past, good old days, happy times

Common expressions: 'how beautiful it was in those days', 'those were the 'golden times'.

State of mind: a nostalgic person, stuck in the past, absence of spirit, sadness or nostalgia in the eyes.

Examples of situations where we might consider this remedy: any state of nostalgia and regret after a transition from happy times, when a person spent time with people they love, in places where it was beautiful, in happy periods of life, in a period where that person, circumstances or place is no longer there:

- mourning a loved one or friend who has moved to another city or passed away
- regret because your favourite restaurant has closed
- longing for times past, when the president or government in the country changes
- moving to another country with nostalgia for the homeland
- change of job while at the same time missing the previous job
- mourning a lost sports career after injury
- when older people long for moments of their youth
- regretting failed pregnancies while thinking about those pregnancies and unborn children
- grieving for an ex-partner after a breakup
- nostalgia and frequent thinking about places the person has previously travelled to

- retired people longing for their active working days
- people who are adults and employed longing for their days as students
- married people with nostalgia for the days when they were single
- an employed person longing for the times when they were occupied with their favourite hobby and who no longer have time for a hobby
- lamenting over an old car or house

Examples of people who might need this flower remedy: widowed people, divorced people, the elderly, emigrants and all those who mourn the good times of the past.

Positive outcome of the application of this flower remedy: a person will be able to focus on the present and discover joyful things and moments in the present.

Note: this flower remedy will not make a person forget the past, forget dear people who are no longer present, but will only make it easier to deal in the present with the fact that these people, places or times are no longer there – all without sadness, grief or nostalgia.

Examples from practice

I once helped a lady whose husband had passed away. She was still young and she was left alone with small children. She had a hard time dealing with the fact that he was no longer there. Both she and the children now have only memories of the good times when they were all together.

There were several types of flower remedies in their bottles, from those for sadness and shock to flower remedies for adjustment, but it was very important that they also took Honeysuckle. Nostalgia and memories of a lost loved one and the happy times when they were together kept them stuck in grief.

The children responded well to the flower remedies and very quickly grasped which flower remedies were used for which condition. They learned to mix Bach flower remedies themselves. The girl, who until then had suffered greatly for her father and was shy, turned into a cheerful girl full of self-confidence. This is an example of a whole family taking their health and their lives into their own hands while consciously working on resolving their feelings and traumas.

Another example of how Honeysuckle can help with the loss of a loved one was one of my clients whose wife had passed away. Although several years had passed since that unfortunate event, and he had moved to another place of residence with his children, he often walked to the apartment where they lived, after which he would return in tears. Every reminder of their life together was painful for him. So he came for help at every anniversary (engagement, marriage, her birthday). Every slightest reminder of her was painful to him. The combination of remedies, which included Honeysuckle, helped him build a new life. He found a wonderful wife who is now a good mother to his children and whom the children adore. This extremely sad story, as a result of the application of Bach flower remedies, became a story of a happy new family.

But there are also Honeysuckle stories that are not necessarily sad in character. Honeysuckle is my favourite Bach flower. It has an unusual appearance and a bright cyclamen colour. When I place it in the context of the meaning of the remedy, the appearance of the flower acquires a deeper meaning for me. To me personally, it looks like a hand in which a person holds something – some memory, some person, some happy times.

I also often wander off into the Honeysuckle state, into fond memories. My husband and I get carried away in the Honeysuckle state if we watch some travel or culinary shows about the countries we have visited. And then I remember everything and I feel as if I was there at that moment, as if I was seeing, hearing, smelling and feeling everything again … The magical Indian cuisine, the *masala* tea, the *gulab jamun* dessert and the amusing continuous sounds of car horns. The beauties of the Sicilian landscape, climbing the magnificent volcano Etna and various desserts made from pistachios. Walks along the Spanish coast and beautiful sandy beaches overlooking Gibraltar. The dazzling lights of New York and a boat ride to the Statue of Liberty. Warm sea and purple skies in Miami. *Priganice* in Montenegro prepared by my best friend Lidija. Yes, food can also steer us into a state of nostalgia. For me, these are unusual and delicious delicacies that I do not have in Zagreb, and I tried them once in a distant city. Sometimes certain dishes take me back to my youth – like Lika soup on Gacka, served with warm bread and butter, or the legendary *rizi-bizi* (rice with peas) that Štefica used to cook for me, as well as the polenta with milk prepared by my mother.

When we remember those times, we look with nostalgia at the old photos we took, and we remember the delicious food and beautiful landscapes – that's the Honeysuckle state. And when you fall into that state, it really is a nice feeling. But do take this flower remedy if this happens to you too often, and if it interferes with your daily activities and business tasks.

> *Remember: Honeysuckle helps us to remember the past without sadness and pain, and to exist in the present without mourning the loss of times past. This flower remedy teaches us gratitude for the times we have lived through, with the people we loved, in the places where we were happy. We realise that these experiences have brought us to where we are today and help us find happiness again where we are now.*

HORNBEAM
Carpinus betulus

Dr. Bach's final description of the flower remedy: 'For those who feel that they have not sufficient strength, mentally or physically, to carry the burden of life placed upon them; the affairs of every day seem too much for them to accomplish, though they generally succeed in fulfilling their task. For those who believe that some part, of mind or body, needs to be strengthened before they can easily fulfil their work.'

Group of remedies: for uncertainty

Key words for recognising the remedy: lethargy, sluggishness, laziness, lack of will or strength

Common expressions: 'I don't feel like it', 'I wish I didn't have to go to work', 'if only I didn't have to do this now', 'I don't have the strength to get out of bed now', 'I don't have the strength to do it.'

State of mind: people not inclined to engage in physical or mental work, people without energy, people in lazy state, mentally exhausted and tired people.

Examples of situations where we might consider this remedy: Monday morning, morning before work, procrastination.

Examples of people who might need this flower remedy: students who procrastinate when studying for an exam, people who need to get up early for work, going to work or school on Monday mornings after the weekend – when they don't have the strength to get up and get going.

Positive outcome of the application of this flower remedy: the person will find the strength and will to get out of bed and attend to the task at hand; they will have a lot of energy and will do even more work than they needed to. There is a rush of energy and motivation to do things that have been delayed for a long time.

The difference between Hornbeam and Olive – fatigue:

Hornbeam is a state of fatigue <u>before work</u>, from the very thought of the job to be done. It is a mental fatigue, which is accompanied by a feeling of heaviness in the body and a feeling of inability to get going and do the task that needs to be done. A person has a feeling that she or he does not have the strength to perform a job or task.

Olive is a state of fatigue <u>after work</u>. It is the physical fatigue that follows a job done or an exhausting illness, unlike Hornbeam whose fatigue occurs <u>before</u> a job is even started.

Examples from practice

Once a client came to me for a consultation and asked me to recommend remedies for her husband, who was constantly putting off some obligations that he needed to fulfil. I recommended Hornbeam flower remedy, and here are her impressions after he started using this flower remedy: 'I asked Ana to help me because I needed remedies for my husband, because he never finishes things; hence, everything remains unfinished. He started taking them and began literally carrying closets on his back, something that had needed to be done over a year ago! A real miracle!!!'

I can confirm that I feel the same effect when I take this flower remedy. I remember very well one situation when I was still teaching accounting. That day I didn't feel like giving a lecture at all, and I knew I had to because the students were waiting for me in the auditorium and I could not postpone the lecture. To ease my 'anguish', I took Hornbeam flower remedy and set out to give the lecture. I held the lecture with ease, not noticing how the flower remedy had actually lifted my energy and mood. It wasn't until I got home and started to tidy up the closet, which was by no means in my plan before (and I had been putting it off for weeks), that I realised what was going on and I burst out laughing! Not only had this flower remedy given me the energy and motivation to do what I had to do that day, but I also had the energy for the extra task of tidying up the closet, which without taking this flower remedy would certainly not have been on my schedule that day.

 Remember: Hornbeam flower remedy gives us the mental and physical strength to easily and happily fulfil the obligations ahead of us – without fatigue, without whining and complaining, and without delay.

IMPATIENS

Impatiens royleii[19]

Dr. Bach's description of the flower: '... beautiful mauve flower, Impatiens, which grows along the sides of some of the Welsh streams[20]...'

Dr. Bach's final description of the flower remedy: 'Those who are quick in thought and action and who wish all things to be done without hesitation or delay. When ill they are anxious for a hasty recovery. They find it very difficult to be patient with people who are slow, as they consider it wrong and a waste of time, and they will endeavour to make such people quicker in all ways. They often prefer to work and think alone, so that they can do everything at their own speed.'

Description from *The Story of the Travellers* (1934): Indication: 'Impatiens, too, well knew the pathway home, so well that he was impatient with those less speedy than himself.' Positive outcome: 'Impatiens knows no hurry, but lingers among the hindmost to keep their pace ...'.

Group of remedies: for loneliness

Key words for recognising the remedy: impatience, haste, irritability, tempo

Common expressions: 'Hurry up!', 'How long does it take you to do it?', 'Oh, you are so slow!', 'Give it to me, I'll do it faster!', 'I'm leaving, I cannot wait for you any more!'

Personality type: accelerated, impatient, nervous, stomping, eating fast, walking fast.

---

[19] Modern name: *Impatiens glandulifera.*
[20] Bach first found the flower *Impatiens glandulifera* growing by a stream in the Abergavenny area of Wales in 1928.

Examples of situations where we might consider this remedy:

- waiting impatiently for results of medical examinations
- waiting in line at a store, bank or post office while the people in front seem to take for ever
- flying on an airplane when a person is impatient to land
- a woman who is impatient to give birth
- a husband who is impatient to wait for his wife to give birth
- waiting for a flight at the airport and wishing it would hurry up
- impatience to see results of a treatment and the effects of a therapy
- impatience to see a person on a diet start losing weight
- impatience when driving a car
- children's impatience at school, who cannot wait for classes to finish and to go home
- looking forward to a birthday, Christmas or a holiday and wishing it were here already!

Examples of people who might need this flower remedy: people impatient in traffic, people who cannot stand waiting in line or at a bank or store.

Positive outcome of the application of this flower remedy: a person develops tolerance for other people's pace, is ready to stand patiently in line, and is ready to wait for others to complete the task without being impatient.

Examples from practice

You've probably experienced this before at some point and seen it with your own eyes – a person speeding, honking their horn (except in India where honking is perfectly normal in traffic), cursing and overtaking other cars. Or you are standing in line at a store at the checkout and the person behind you complains about how slow the cashier is and complains that they have been waiting for too long. Or have you ever waited in line at a fast-food restaurant, and you waited four minutes instead of the expected two, and immediately commented that it was inadmissible for you to wait that long?

These are all situations in which Impatiens reacts with anger – complaining, protesting, rebelling, shouting and sometimes exploding, thus provoking an argument or a fight.

Impatiens clients are also easy to identify in a consultation. They are usually upset if they need to wait a few minutes for me to complete a consultation with a previous client. Or they hurry me from the very beginning of the consultation and remark that they are in a hurry and that we should make the conversation as short as possible. Some keep looking at the clock due to impatience, or they keep tapping their foot. Some, on the other hand, are not so impatient during the consultations themselves, but declare that they are impatient.

Still, the person may not be visibly impatient, but they haven't the patience to wait a certain amount of time for the therapy to start working. So some clients give up using homeopathic remedies or Bach flower remedies if they do not feel instant relief and withdrawal of symptoms, forgetting that the disease also did not appear overnight, hence the symptoms cannot disappear overnight. Again, it is all about impatience.

I personally take Impatiens when I am teaching and I have limited time to transfer all the planned teachings. With this flower remedy, I don't look at the clock constantly and I am not stressed out because of time limitations, and I am not impatient about wanting to talk about everything there is in my lesson plan, but I teach in a relaxed and calm manner, so when the lecture is over, I see that I managed to do everything in time and in the set time frame. This remedy gives me a good sense of time and keeps my tempo, which suits both me and the group, so I am well coordinated with the group. I would also recommend this remedy to students and pupils taking a test when there is a time limit, if they usually feel impatient and hastened while taking a test. Impatiens will give you a good sense of time to solve everything in given time.

Additional advice: For those who are always late and slow, add Chestnut Bud so that they can learn from their mistakes. For those who are always in a hurry, and are nervous and angry about other people's slowness, add Impatiens to their mix to calm down their impulse to explode.

Remember: Impatiens flower remedy gives us calmness and patience when performing our daily activities, and reduces impatience when waiting. It teaches us tolerance towards other people's pace of fulfilling obligations and actions, and we become more ready for teamwork.

LARCH

Larix europaea[21]

Dr. Bach's final description of the flower remedy: 'For those who do not consider themselves as good or capable as those around them, who expect failure, who feel that they will never be a success, and so do not venture or make a strong enough attempt to succeed.'

Group of remedies: for despondency or despair

Key words for recognising the remedy: lack of self-confidence (sometimes due to feeling that one has lack of knowledge or lack of ability to perform)

Common expressions: 'I don't know to do that', 'I cannot do it', 'I'm not good enough for this job position', 'I don't have the capacity for it', 'I don't have enough self-confidence to take over this duty.'

Personality type: insecure, but can either hide or openly show their insecurity.

Examples of situations where we might consider this remedy: any situation in which a person doubts their own ability to do the task at hand:

- they doubt their knowledge and abilities, and do not apply for a job vacancy
- they doubt their acquired knowledge and give up competing at a school competition
- they doubt their performance and give up competing at a sports competition

---

[21] Modern name: *Larix decidua*.

Their reaction might be in one of the following forms:

- does not accept offered opportunities, with the explanation that they do not have the capacity to do so (admits doubt in their abilities or knowledge)

- accepts the offered opportunity, but due to doubt in their abilities gives up and states that they cannot do it (admits doubt in their abilities or knowledge)

- accepts the offered opportunity, but due to the fear that they will not know or be able to complete the accepted assignment, they develop fever, a tummy bug or some other problem, and are happy that they are freed from the task due to illness (lack of self-confidence remains hidden from others)

- accepts the offered opportunity, but for fear that they will not know or be able to do it, uses lies and reports that they have a fever, tummy bug or other problems due to which they cannot do the task (lack of self-confidence remains hidden from others)

- recommends another person who is available to do the task for them, noting that this is a great opportunity for that person and that they should be given the opportunity (lack of self-confidence remains hidden from others)

Examples of people who might need this flower remedy: performers before a performance, pupils and students before an exam, employees in a new job or taking on a new role, teenagers, etc. – if they lack self-confidence.

Positive outcome of the application of this flower remedy: the person will have more confidence to accept a task or job, and will believe in their own abilities, knowledge and talents.

The difference between Larch and Crab Apple – lack of self-confidence:

Larch has a lack of self-confidence because they believe that they do not have the necessary qualities and knowledge to do a job, or to perform a task.

Crab Apple has a lack of self-confidence because they think they are not pretty enough, skinny enough, attractive enough, and have a problem with their appearance.

Therefore, the root cause of Larch's lack of self-confidence is in the thinking that they lag behind in their mental and physical abilities, or lack the talent or ability to do a job, while Crab Apple's reason for lack of self-confidence is dissatisfaction with their own appearance.

Larch says: <u>I am not able to</u> ... do this well, pass the exam, etc.

Crab Apple says: <u>I am not</u> ... beautiful, skinny, attractive, tall, etc.

Examples from practice

Here is an example and the impressions of a client of mine, after I recommended Larch flower remedy to her:

'When I started my own business and I had to perform and present products in a country where I am a foreigner, I felt inferior, nervous, incompetent, and I also had no experience in that. Then Ana recommended the flower remedies to me and in a very short time I felt superior, and I could not wait to start business negotiations and to sign the contracts.'

I also recommended Larch flower remedy to a young teacher who, after graduating from college, got her first job as a primary school teacher. She was nervous about the first day of the PTA meeting, how she would present herself in front of all the parents. She also thought about how she would cope with her older and more experienced colleagues. After just two days of using this flower remedy, she called me feeling great and full of confidence. She no longer doubted her abilities and did all the tasks well, including her first parent-teacher meeting.

Remember: Larch gives us faith in our own abilities, knowledge and talents. It teaches us to accept compliments for completed tasks and acquired knowledge. It gives us the courage to accept the tasks that others have entrusted to us with confidence, and helps us to do the work ahead of us in a relaxed and self-confident way.

MIMULUS

Mimulus luteus[22]

Dr. Bach's description of the flower: '… Mimulus, found growing on the sides of the crystal streams …', '… a beautiful plant called MIMULUS: rather like Musk. Some summers it grows in the stream at Ewelme, which runs alongside the road.'

---

[22] Modern name: *Mimulus guttatus*.

Dr. Bach's final description of the flower remedy: 'Fear of worldly things, illness, pain, accidents, poverty, of dark, of being alone, of misfortune. The fears of everyday life. These people quietly and secretly bear their dread; they do not freely speak of it to others.'

Dr. Bach's lecture on this flower remedy: 'The second kind of fear is more common: and is the one which applies to everyday life. The ordinary fears so many of us get. Fear of accidents, fear of illness, fear of a complaint getting worse, fear of the dark, of being alone, of burglars, or fire, of poverty, of animals, of other people and so on. Fears of definite things, whether there be any reason or not.'

Description from *The Story of the Travellers* (1934): Indication: 'Mimulus began to be afraid, afraid that they had lost the road.' Positive outcome: 'Mimulus can know no fear ....'.

Group of remedies: for fear

Key words for recognising the remedy: fear, shyness

Common expressions: 'I am afraid', 'I am shy', 'I am embarrassed.'

Personality type: fearful, shy, quiet, withdrawn person. Possibly has a low tone of voice, looks at the floor, stands in the corner, bites his/her nails.

Examples of situations where we might consider this remedy: fear of dentists, doctors, blood sampling, flying, dogs, diseases, death, etc.

Examples of people who might need this flower remedy: shy person, shy kids at school, performers who suffer from stage fright before a public performance, those with known fears that can be named.

Positive outcome of the application of this flower remedy: the person will have more courage and will not be afraid of illness, darkness, flying, etc. A shy person will feel more comfortable in the company of other people, in society, before a public appearance.

The difference between Mimulus and Larch – fear of public appearance or exam:

Mimulus is afraid in front of an audience because of their shyness or is afraid of the audience's reaction to their performance. Mimulus is afraid before an exam because they fear the reaction of their parents or teacher if they do not know all the answers or if they get a bad grade. Mimulus naturally has stage fright, but because of shyness, not a lack of self-confidence.

Larch is afraid before a public appearance or exam because they think they do not know enough, that they haven't learned enough or that they cannot do something.

It is possible and desirable to combine Mimulus and Larch in one bottle before a public performance or an exam if there are elements for the application of both flower remedies.

Difference in the use of Mimulus flower remedy for acute state and personality type:

- Mimulus type is shy and we will recommend Mimulus to overcome that shyness (remedy for the type of person).

- Mimulus type is shy and afraid of public appearances that are soon to take place. She or he needs Mimulus flower remedy both for shyness (remedy for the type of person) and for fear of public appearance (flower remedy for the state of mind).

- The person is not a Mimulus type and is not shy, but is a very good speaker and performer. He or she usually performs in front of an audience, but has fear and nervousness before a public performance. They need Mimulus because it is an acute state (remedy for the state of mind), although they are not a Mimulus type.

Examples from practice

'My first type'

You wouldn't believe it, but in my student booklet, throughout the first four grades of elementary school, it was written regularly, 'Ana is quiet, calm and withdrawn. She needs to be encouraged to express herself. She does not like to read aloud or answer orally.' Yes, that was my first type, of which there is no trace today. Today I have no problem giving a lecture even in front of five hundred people. Today I feel best when I teach, when I speak in front of an audience, when I am on the podium. Unfortunately, my parents did not give me Mimulus flower remedy, but I overcame that type or state on my own over time. If only I had had Mimulus! I would have been spared so many troubles.

Even Dr. Rajan Sankaran, whom I consider the most influential homeopath of our time, writes in his autobiography, *Dog Yogi, Banjan Tree*, that as a child he was very withdrawn and shy, and did not like to stand out. Today he gives lectures all over the world.

The same story is told by Anita Moorjani in her book *What if This is Heaven?*, where she writes about how she just wanted to become invisible, so that no one would notice her, and further describes that although her mother tirelessly tried to get her out of her armour, most of her youth she remained very shy and withdrawn. Today, she is also a successful speaker and tells her story around the world.

In his book *The Sensation in Homeopathy*, Dr. Sankaran states that people who do not have self-confidence, or are afraid of public speaking, have the potential to become excellent speakers. That these are two sides of the same coin – fear and courage, that is, great shyness and a great gift of speech.

These examples show us that the gift of speech is sometimes given to shy people, who have the task of overcoming this shyness in order to spread their ideas and teachings further.

Therefore, the examples I have previously given present an accurate description of children who are in need of this flower remedy. These are shy, quiet, and withdrawn children, who like to be in the shadows and do not like to speak in public, in front of others. If you have such a child or know such a child or person, help them overcome that state or type and recommend Mimulus flower remedy. You will quickly notice changes and they will start to open up more and more in their communication with others.

Other applications of this flower remedy in my practice have been most commonly intended to help with fear of disease, fear of the dark, fear of flying on an airplane, fear of dentists, fear of surgery, fear of exams, fear of public appearance, and other similar fears.

Do you remember the story of the Wizard of Oz, when the Cowardly Lion asked for courage? That lion needed Mimulus flower remedy. This is the flower remedy that gives courage to the timid and provides self-confidence to the shy.

Remember: Mimulus flower remedy will help us gain courage in dealing with known fears, and will help us overcome shyness and fear of public speaking. This flower remedy will make the little mouse turn into a brave lion.

MUSTARD

Sinapis arvensis

Dr. Bach's final description of the flower remedy: 'Those who are liable to times of gloom, or even despair, as though a cold dark cloud overshadowed them and hid the light and the joy of life. It may not be possible to give any reason or explanation for such attacks. Under these conditions it is almost impossible to appear happy or cheerful.'

Group of remedies: for insufficient interest in present circumstances

Key words for recognising the remedy: mood swings, depression for no reason

Common expressions: 'as if a grey cloud hovers over me', 'I am not in a good mood, but do not know why', 'I got out of the wrong side of the bed this morning.'

State of mind: shifting and gloomy mood.

Examples of situations where we might consider this remedy: malaise or depression for no reason.

Examples of people who might need this flower remedy: women with PMS or in menopause, pregnant women, all those who experience shifting moods or depressed mood for no real reason.

Positive outcome of the application of this flower remedy: the person will see the beauty of the life they live and view positively every situation they face. The person will experience a surge of positive energy.

Examples from practice

This is the flower remedy I tried last out of all 38 flower remedies. I was doing homework for my Level 1 education about Bach flower remedies. The assignment required me to describe how I felt in the situation when I took the Mustard flower remedy. It was then that I realised I had never actually tried this remedy. I closed my homework, went to my bedroom where I kept my Bach flower remedies box, took Mustard flower remedy to try it, and went to the kitchen to wash the dishes. After about ten minutes, I felt a rush of happiness. My husband was watching TV at the time, and I suddenly started explaining to him how beautiful our lives are, how beautiful our children are and how happy I am. And then I sat down and finished my homework. I realised how Mustard flower remedy works. It is there to show us the beauty of our lives and all those things we should be thankful for, at the same time removing worries and negative feelings and thoughts, which have no place because there is no real reason for any negativity.

So I recommended Mustard flower remedy to a client who was always focused on some gloomy thoughts, and at the same time did not see how beautiful and amazing her children were. She always saw only their flaws; for example, that they did not wash the dishes. But she did not see that she raised wonderful adults and responsible young people. Mustard's job was to show her things to be grateful for, instead of ones to complain about.

One of my dear clients and friends, who has achieved great professional success, and is highly esteemed in her business and social circles, always used to find something to complain about. Thus, she would get angry at the craftsmen, the people she met that day, etc. In addition, she was suffering from mood swings because she was entering menopause. Bach flower remedies bottles, which always contain Mustard, complement her every day and she loves to use them. This Mustard flower remedy always calms her down and she considers it to be her main flower remedy for 'emergencies'.

> *Remember: Mustard flower remedy helps us disperse the dark clouds that hover over our lives, and makes us realise all the beauty and joy of the life we live, without sadness, depression or mood swings.*

OAK

Quercus pedunculata[23]

Dr. Bach's final description of the flower remedy: 'For those who are struggling and fighting strongly to get well, or in connection with the affairs of their daily life. They will go on trying one thing after another, though their case may seem hopeless. They will fight on. They are discontented with themselves if illness interferes with their duties or helping others. They are brave people, fighting against great difficulties, without loss of hope or effort.'

Description from *The Story of the Travellers* (1934): Indication: 'Oak, on the other hand, though feeling all was lost and that they would never again see the sunshine said, "I

---

[23] Modern name: *Quercus robur*.

shall struggle on to the very last", and he did in a wild way.' Positive outcome: 'Oak stands steadfast in the strongest gale …'.

Group of remedies: for despondency or despair

Key words for recognising the remedy: strength, responsibility, I must

Common expressions: 'I have to do it', 'I don't have time to rest', 'I have a responsibility to others', 'Who will do it if I don't?'

Personality type: this is the most durable and strongest type of remedy. Oak does not give up and works beyond the limits of their endurance. The Oak person does not rest and does not waste time on nonsense, but is always busy. She or he is highly responsible because they know they have to feed their family, pay salaries to employees or run a business, company, state, etc. responsibly. They can be exhausted by work and ignore the symptoms of illness or weakness. Oak never gives up and never loses hope. Oak has a motto: 'Work, work and only work.' Work to the last breath.

Examples of situations where we might consider this remedy: any exaggeration connected with work, with a great sense of responsibility, and where one's own body and health are abused:

- exhaustion from overwork (working beyond one's limits of endurance)

- not going on vacation

- not taking breaks during working hours

- working day and night

- working during illness

- caring for children, or if one is a doctor for patients, when the person themself is ill

Even though some other remedy types can overwork (Vervain, Impatience, Elm, etc.), the keynote to recognise in Oak is her or his sense of endurance, struggle and effort, refusal to give in, a slow and steady strength. This is different from Vervain who might be overly enthusiastic about some project and working overtime, or Impatiens who is overworking as he is taking on the workload of his colleagues who were executing their tasks too slowly, so Impatiens took these on to himself. And please see the section on Elm to differentiate Oak and Elm regarding overworking.

Examples of people who might need this flower remedy: directors, business owners, single parents, a parent with many children – if they are feeling an enormous sense of responsibility where they won't allow themselves to give in.

Positive outcome of the application of this flower remedy: an Oak person will not always realise that they need help and will not seek help in order to work less, because these are responsible and strong people who can bear a lot on their backs. But when they realise that they have reached the limits of their physical endurance, they might some day seek help. Then the flower remedy will not remove their positive qualities, such as responsibility and diligence, nor reduce their endurance, but will work to make the person recognise when the body has really reached the limits of endurance, and then lie down and rest. The positive outcome of applying Oak flower remedy is that the person will begin to listen to their body and recognise the body's signals when it seeks rest. An Oak person may, for the first time, take a day off, take a walk or rest, go home from work when they are sick instead of working through sickness as usual. In doing so, they will learn to delegate work, develop more confidence that co-workers and employees will do a good job while they are away, and will realise that their work will not suffer if they take a little rest.

Important: not a single remedy will nullify the positive qualities that a person possesses, but will only balance and eradicate the negative traits. Likewise, flower remedies cannot be taken to develop some quality that we do not have. For example, we cannot give Oak flower remedy to a person who is an artist and expect that person to become a leader or director if they do not already carry those characteristics and qualities within them.

'The Story of the Oak Tree', by Dr. Bach (1934)

'One day, and not very long ago, a man was leaning against an oak tree in an old park in Surrey, and he heard what the oak tree was thinking. Now that sounds a very funny thing, but trees do think, you know, and some people can understand what they are thinking.

This old oak tree, and it was a very old oak tree, was saying to itself, "How I envy those cows in the meadow that can walk about the field, and here I am; and everything around so beautiful, so wonderful, the sunshine and the breezes and the rain and yet I am rooted to the spot."

And years afterwards the man found that in the flowers of the oak tree was a great power, the power to heal a lot of sick people, and so he collected the flowers of the oak trees and made them into medicines, and lots and lots of people were healed and made well again.

Some time after this on a hot summer's afternoon, the man was lying on the edge of a cornfield very nearly asleep, and he heard a tree thinking, as some people can hear trees think. The tree was speaking to itself very quietly, and it was saying, "I don't any longer envy the cows who can walk about the meadows, because I can go to all the four quarters of the world to heal the people who are ill": and the man looked up and found that it was an oak tree thinking.'

Examples from practice

Do you know a person who works, works and works, all the way to the point of exhaustion?

According to Nora Weeks, that is how Dr. Bach worked: 'He worked non-stop, without rest, until he felt so bad that he fainted in the lab. His great determination not to give up in the face of his weaknesses, as long as there was so much work to be done and as long as there were so many people in need of help, kept him active for a time, until he fainted in July 1917, as result of severe bleeding.'[24] In the same book, Nora continues giving similar examples, of how he behaved after a major surgery, thus confirming the thesis that Dr. Bach could be the Oak type: 'Although he was still exhausted and could barely walk, he returned to the hospital laboratory, where he managed the entire department for several weeks. In an instant he got so immersed in that experience that he completely forgot about time, and he worked day and night, so much so that the light from the window of his laboratory was said to be "a light that never goes out".'[25]

---

[24] Nora Weeks, *The Medical Discoveries of Edward Bach Physician,* The C.W. Daniel Company Limited (1975), p. 21.
[25] Ibid. p. 22.

A person in an Oak state or a person who is an Oak type will put work ahead of everything, including their health. This sense of responsibility does not allow them to rest even on days when they feel exhausted or sick.

Interestingly, this flower remedy had its turn in my writing today, when I stayed at home because I have a cold with a sore throat. I am laughing out loud right now, thinking how everything happens so I can convey to you the power of every remedy and present them in the best light possible. My first impression was that I actually balanced the Oak flower remedy, because I did stay at home today, instead of going to work and working while sick. And then I start laughing because I realise I am not resting but writing a book! Here is a typical example of the need to take Oak flower remedy. So, this is how a person in the Oak state or a person who is the Oak type thinks. After getting some sleep, resting, I started working on the book in the afternoon. Oak does not rest if there is a job they can do.

My dad used to tell me when I was a teenager, 'We can always find a job we can do.' So on one occasion he gave me a task. He told me to tidy up my wardrobe. I took all the things out of the closet and arranged everything neatly. I proudly showed him how I had arranged everything, hoping that I would now be able to go out with my friends. But he then intended to teach me an important lesson. He said: 'You did a great job. Everything is very nicely folded. But now you take everything out of the closet, fold it again and put it all back.' I looked at him in astonishment, and he said, 'You see, we can always find something to do if we want to work!'

Yes, my father instilled in me the qualities of Oak flower remedy. That is, it is obvious that I already had those qualities in myself. But, because of my Oak nature, I almost broke down twice in my life under the pressure of obligations and responsibilities. And then my Oak flower remedy did the thing and taught me what the word 'BALANCE' means. It has been the main word in my dictionary ever since! Oak flower remedy taught me to find balance! I realised that apart from having work and responsibilities, it is equally important to rest, that it is equally important to have a hobby, that it is extremely important to find enough time for family and the people who are important to you. That it is important to enjoy life. That it is important to go on vacation, in nature, take a walk, sit down with my husband for coffee. That sometimes it is important to just be lazy!

Once upon a time, my father maintained such a balance. Fishing provided this balance for him and we spent every free weekend or vacation on the River Gacka. The River Gacka and the war-torn Hotel Gacka often lead me into the state of Honeysuckle flower remedy (thinking about past happy times). Those were indeed beautiful and happy times. As a baby, I began to crawl there for the first time. There I ran merrily and happily in nature. I spent almost all my childhood vacations and holidays there. There I walked and observed the beautiful forget-me-nots along the river. Because of these memories, forget-me-not is still my favourite flower and adorns the logo of my company. Back then, my dad had a hobby, and set aside time for field trips and family trips. Unfortunately, after the founding of his company, his imbalance of Oak flower remedy made him forget about hobbies, free time, pleasures, aimless relaxing walks around the city … and over time he became a tired and worried person with poor health. Since then he has achieved numerous exceptional successes and attained recognition in his life, but at the expense of his health and balance. He stopped going on vacation. He travels only if the trip has a business purpose. He does not like holidays and non-working days because, for him, it is a waste of time. He still works and is not familiar with the word 'retirement'. I am personally grateful to him today for the lessons I have learned by observing his model of work and life. He showed me by his example that this is not my way or model of functioning, even though I have my own companies. His story taught both me and my husband to always pay close attention to the balance between work and the things that make us happy. And that work can be neither an excuse nor a substitute for rest and the relaxing time we need to spend with a partner and family.

To summarise the effect of Oak flower remedy: the opposite of the word balance is imbalance. An imbalance. And this imbalance can best be shown with a description of the negative state of Oak flower remedy. A person who has not balanced their Oak type or Oak state abuses their body because of responsibility and work. Impaired health is the result of their diligence, dedication to work and responsibility. An Oak who is out of balance puts responsibility first, even before his or her health.

But here it is also necessary to point out the tremendously positive sides of the Oak person. When the positive sides of Oak flower remedy prevail, this is a person you admire for their strength. This is a person who will never let you down because they have an extremely developed sense of responsibility. It is a person who will find, somewhere deep inside, the strength to endure, no matter how hard it may be. And they will never complain or whine. They carry their burden like a stoic and will carry your burden as well without discussion.

Here I can give the example of my friend Maja, whom I have known since my earliest childhood. She grew up with a sick older sister, who died young, tragically, as a result of an accident. Maja played sports most of her youth and trained hard. As an adult, she showed her Oak strenght by caring for her seriously ill mother for years, helping her father, despite having two young children, and despite a demanding job where she works with children with disabilities. Her commitment to her mother, whom she regularly brought to my centre for consultations, enabled her mother to have a better quality of life. She selflessly gave her love and attention, despite the fact that it was not at all easy for her and that she barely managed to accomplish everything during the day. I never heard her complain. She never asked for help for herself. Just for her mother. Whenever I offered her help, she would always say, 'I'm great, I have it easy. It is important that my mother gets better.'

This is the power of Oak flower remedy that we admire over and over again. It is wonderful to be an Oak person. Such people are our role models and pillars of our stability when the ground slips from under our feet. All that matters is that Oak stays in balance, that they find enough time for themselves as well, because their batteries also need to be charged. People need to rest and get enough sleep. With an awareness of the importance of caring for your physical body, it is wonderful to be an Oak type, because it is the most powerful type of all the personalities in Bach's system of remedies.

 Remember: Oak flower remedy helps us strike a balance between business and our own leisure time – between our time for work and our time for rest. Oak teaches us to listen to the signals of our body, and to take more care of our health and body.

OLIVE

Olea europaea

Dr. Bach's final description of the flower remedy: 'Those who have suffered much mentally or physically and are so exhausted and weary that they feel they have no more strength to make any effort. Daily life is hard work for them, without pleasure.'

Group of remedies: for insufficient interest in present circumstances

Key words for recognising the remedy: tiredness, exhaustion

Common expressions: 'I am too tired', 'I am dead on my feet', 'I can barely stand on my feet.'

State of mind: exhaustion, weakness, no energy.

Examples of situations where we might consider this remedy: exhaustion and fatigue after work or after illness, persons who are tired during or after a journey, during or after childbirth.

Examples of people who might need this flower remedy: people who are tired in some of the following situations or states: working overtime, working night shifts, pregnant women, women who just gave birth, parents of young children, patients suffering from severe or debilitating illnesses, athletes after strenuous training or competition, workers who do hard physical work.

Positive outcome of the application of this flower remedy: revitalisation of mind and body.

Similarities and differences with other flower remedies – for fatigue:

Olive is a state of tiredness <u>after</u> work, while Hornbeam is a state of fatigue from the very thought of work, even <u>before</u> any effort is made.

Elm and Oak can also be overworked and exhausted. Elm is exhausted from too many commitments and overloaded with obligations, and Oak is exhausted because she rarely rests, as she has a high sense of duty and responsibility. So we can also add Olive flower remedy to these people's personal bottle of flower remedies.

A person in Olive state wants to rest. Either they fall asleep but not even sleep can help them recuperate after fatigue or illness, or they have a lot of responsibilities so are not yet able to lie down and rest or sleep.

Elm cannot rest because they have too many obligations, but they want to rest and give up under the burden of obligations.

Oak has no time to rest and does not give up, but tries to endure until they have drained the last atom of strength in their body.

Olive flower remedy can hence be perfect for people in Elm state, or people who are Oak type or are in Oak state.

Note: Olive flower remedy does not have the effect of coffee or energy drinks.

This flower remedy will, in some states, give you the strength to endure and finish the task at hand, and in other situations will make you go to bed and rest. The flower remedies will always do what is best for you at a certain point, so listen to what your body is telling you after you take this flower remedy. If you still feel tired and exhausted after taking Olive flower remedy, it may be a signal that you urgently need to sleep and rest. So lie down, rest and sleep!

Important note: if you are tired from driving or operating machinery, do not take Olive flower remedy as a substitute for rest. Do not drive while you are tired and exhausted, but stop the vehicle and rest, and only then continue the journey.

Examples from practice

One client was going through the recovery phase after a difficult gastric cancer operation, had a poor appetite, and was in a tortured and weakened physical condition. He successively took Bach's Olive flower remedy to physically recover from illness, surgery and chemotherapy. He soon got stronger, started eating better and recovered.

However, I have also recommended Olive flower remedy for physical exhaustion to my clients who are athletes, if they feel tired and exhausted. And I give Olive flower remedy to my son Ante, who is a handball goalkeeper, after hard training and tournaments, if he is feeling worn out and exhausted.

People who do heavy physical work at work, at home or in the field should definitely take Olive flower remedy if they feel exhausted at the end of the day. Even hard mental work can be very exhausting for a person. A friend of mine who is a finance director in a large company, after a work day that requires high concentration and responsibility, makes sure to use Olive flower remedy as she feels extremely exhausted.

Another client, who is a school teacher, after working with the children at the school, comes home where housework awaits her, as well as three children and a husband, and she can barely survive a day without Olive flower remedy. Her husband describes the effect of Olive flower remedy on her as follows: 'My wife is never exhausted. She is cheerful, smiling, goes to bed late, gets up early, loves her husband and always finds time for him. In addition, she washes, cooks – and all with a smile on her face.'

 Remember: Olive flower remedy gives us the strength to do all our daily tasks without fatigue and effortlessly. It revitalises so we can be rested and energetic.

PINE

Pinus sylvestris

Dr. Bach's final description of the flower remedy: 'For those who blame themselves. Even when successful they think that[26] they could have done better, and are never content with their efforts or the results. They are hard-working and suffer much from the faults they attach to themselves. Sometimes if there is any mistake it is due to another, but they will claim responsibility even for that.'

Group of remedies: for despondency or despair

Key words for recognising the remedy: guilt, remorse

Common expressions: 'It's my fault', 'I should have done it better', 'I didn't try hard enough.'

---

[26] The word 'that' is omitted from most later editions of dr. Bach's book.

State of mind or personality type: imaginary or actual guilt or remorse. They take responsibility for something, even if it is someone else's mistake. They are simply convinced that they are to blame.

Examples of situations where we might consider this remedy: any situation in which a person has a sense of guilt, whether the guilt is real or imaginary:

- a person who blames him- or herself and re-examines their mistakes when they learn that their partner is having an affair with another person

- a person who was not promoted and blames her- or himself for, obviously, not doing well enough or trying hard

- a person who, due to work and obligations towards his/her own children and family, cannot devote enough time to a sick parent and feels remorse

- a person who works a lot and has a guilty conscience because they do not spend enough time with their children and partner

- a person is on a business trip while their child has an important performance at school or a sports competition, and they feel guilty because they cannot attend the event

- a person whose loved one has died and now blames himself/herself for not spending enough time with that person while they were alive

Examples of people who might need this flower remedy: children of divorced parents, divorced persons, all persons who did something negative or think they have done something wrong.

Positive outcome of the application of this flower remedy: this flower remedy is not intended to silence a person's sense of remorse for any illegal, unethical or immoral action they are taking, so that they can continue to perform such action without hindrance. Namely, the purpose of all of the remedies is to bring a person into an optimal state. So, after applying this flower remedy, the person will recognise that the things they are doing are bad, they will stop doing them and at the same time they will be free from the feeling of remorse related to those actions. A person who feels guilty, and actually has no reason for that, will be relieved of the guilt and will realise that he or she was not guilty. A typical example of this is the children of divorced parents, who automatically blame themselves and feel that they are the ones who have somehow contributed to their parents' divorce. Another example is a woman who has had a miscarriage and thinks that maybe she herself somehow inadvertently caused it, even though she is on some other level aware that she was mindful about everything and that it was not her fault.

Examples from practice

On one occasion, I had a consultation with a very eminent doctor who was suffering because his patient had died during an operation he was performing and this made him feel very guilty. It bothered him so much that he considered giving up further medical practice. After taking a Bach flower remedies mix containing Pine (for the guilt he felt) and Gorse (for giving up) for a few days, he got rid of the guilt, realised he had done the most he could in the situation, and no longer felt guilty about what had happened. He returned to work and continued to help other people.

Another example concerns a young woman who tried to conceive without success, although there was no medical reason for this. She came to a consultation for help because she had heard that Bach flower remedies could help her. Our conversation led her to her blockage. She felt guilty because she thought that the company she worked for would find it difficult to find a replacement, and she thought that her going on maternity leave would put her employer at a disadvantage. After taking Pine for a few weeks, she was free of the sense of guilt and in two months she got pregnant. She gave birth to a child, went on maternity leave without a sense of guilt, and the company she worked for did not suffer any consequences as she had previously imagined.

A client of mine whose wife passed away was also taking Pine for a long time. He felt tremendous self-reproach and refused to move forward in life and open up to new love. After a few months of using this flower remedy, his emotions were balanced, and he allowed himself happiness and love without guilt and the feeling that he had let his deceased wife down. Today, he is happily married to a woman who took on the role of mother to his children. Together, they cherish the memory of their mother and wife, who left them prematurely. But they themselves believe that she personally, on the other hand, made sure that a person entered their lives who would provide them with the love, care and attention they missed, a person who is simply the best for him and the children.

 Remember: Pine helps us to get rid of guilt and remorse, and to forgive ourselves all our mistakes and blunders. Likewise, this flower remedy implores us to let go of guilt in situations where we have taken someone else's guilt upon ourselves.

RED CHESTNUT

Aesculus carnea

Dr. Bach's final description of the flower remedy: 'For those who find it difficult not to be anxious for other people. Often they have ceased to worry about themselves, but for those of whom they are fond they may suffer much, frequently anticipating that some unfortunate thing may happen to them.'

Dr. Bach's lecture on this flower remedy: '… the fifth kind is the fear for others, especially those dear to us. If they return late, there is the thought that some accident must have happened: if they go for a holiday, the dread that some calamity will befall them. Some illnesses become very serious complaints, and there is great anxiety even for those who are not dangerously ill. Always fearing the worst and always anticipating misfortune for them. The Remedy made from the RED CHESTNUT BLOSSOM, of the tree so well known to all of us, soon removes such fears and helps us to think more normally.'

Group of remedies: for fear

Key words for recognising the remedy: fear and concern for others

Common expression: 'I'm afraid something will happen to him/her.'

Personality type: a person who is not worried about themselves, but for loved ones, who fears that some misfortune may befall them.

Examples of situations where we might consider this remedy:

- a worried parent of a sick child

- a pregnant woman who is concerned about the child she is carrying

- a partner and family who are worried while the woman is in labour

- family members who are worried because the person is ill or undergoing surgery

- a worried parent whose child is leaving only for a field trip or short travel

- a worried parent whose child goes to a nightclub

- a person who is worried when a close person is travelling by plane to a distant country

Examples of people who might need this flower remedy: parents, people who have sick parents, a spouse whose wife is in labour, all who are concerned about the health and well-being of a close person.

Positive outcome of the application of this flower remedy: it is very important to know that this flower remedy will not make you a callous and selfish person when you take it. You will continue to take care for your loved ones, only it will be brought back to normal levels, so that that the worry is not excessive, and will prevent you from imagining black scenarios every time your loved one walks out the door. This means that this flower remedy will help you develop an intuitive feeling that will warn you when to react if your loved ones are in danger, or will calm you down when everything is fine with them.

Examples from practice

To illustrate the power of this flower remedy, I believe it is best to share here my personal examples of how I felt in situations when I was worried for my loved ones.

One time, my son Ante was sick and coughing. He was little, only about two years old. I was very worried because I was always afraid that the cough would get worse and that laryngitis would develop. On that occasion, I stayed up all night, watching him and sitting next to him. I fell asleep early in the morning and he didn't cough that night. Ante woke up in the morning and I was exhausted because I hadn't slept all night. It is amazing that at no point did I remember to take Bach flower remedies, even though I used them extensively at the time. It wasn't until the second night that I remembered Bach flower remedies and took them. I fell asleep normally that night and Ante didn't cough that night either.

This is a typical description of the state in which Red Chestnut flower remedy needs to be taken.

If I had taken Red Chestnut flower remedy that first night, it would have worked in one of these two ways:

- the flower remedy would have calmed me down and the fear would have subsided so I could sleep peacefully; I would then be able to check up on him, if needed, several times during the night, make sure everything was OK with him and go back to sleep
- the flower remedy would have made me feel the need to go to the doctor's office or to sense that it was better to keep an eye on him.

The second example refers precisely to a situation when the flower remedy helps us take sensible action when there might be cause for worry, rather than waste emotional energy on anxiety. In the second story of mine, I was worried because my daughter Eva had had a fever for a few days and also complained of a sore throat. At first I thought I was exaggerating and panicking, thinking her temperature wasn't high and would soon pass. So I took Red Chestnut flower remedy and repeated the dose several times over the course of an hour. But I still felt uneasy, even more so than before, and something urged me to check Eva's condition with the doctor on duty. I went with her to the hospital for an examination and it was established that she had mononucleosis. So, the flower remedy did not calm me down, but helped me take action, rather than waste my emotional energy on anxiety. We received further instructions from the doctor on how to rest, and detailed instructions for her diet, and I was happy that I had reached for the flower remedy.

I have also often given this flower remedy in my practice. I remember this case, when a client sought help for insomnia at my practice. During the conversation, I asked her what her thoughts were when she could not sleep, which is a very important point when determining the most appropriate flower remedy for insomnia. She told me that she was very worried about her husband who had a heart condition and had recently had a stent fitted. He did not rest much, was very active in terms of business and was often away from home. The client confided in me that she does not sleep at night because she is worried about his health and is afraid that one day something will happen to him. I recommended Red Chestnut flower remedy to her, and after taking it she was able to fall asleep normally and sleep peacefully.

Another client was worried about her father, who had heart surgery scheduled for the next week. Because of her apprehension, she could not function normally at work and during the day. After taking Red Chestnut flower remedy, her day was no longer filled with negative thoughts and scenarios about what might happen to him, and she was able to function normally without fear or worry. Her father weathered the operation well and everything was fine, and she realised that she had spent the past week more calmly, that she could devote herself to caring for her father in a quality way, without being upset, scared or negative.

Important note: if you are concerned about the health of people close to you, please refer them or take them to a doctor. It is not advisable to take this flower remedy as a substitute for providing emergency medical care to others.

 Remember: Red Chestnut helps us think positively and to let go of the fears and black premonitions that overwhelm us when we think about the well-being of our loved ones.

ROCK ROSE
Helianthemum vulgare[27]

Dr. Bach's description of the flower: '… beautiful little yellow Rock Rose, which grows so abundantly on our hilly pastures, will give you the courage to win through.'

Dr. Bach's lecture on this flower remedy: 'It is a beautiful thing with a bright yellow flower, it grows on hillsides often

---

[27]   Modern name: *Helianthemum nummularium.*

where the ground is stony or rocky; and a cultivated variety is to be found on rockeries in gardens, though the one growing naturally should always be chosen for healing. This Remedy has had wonderful results, and many an alarming case has been better within minutes or hours of its being given. The key-notes for this Remedy are Panic, terror, great emergency or danger.'

Dr. Bach's final description of the flower remedy: 'The rescue remedy.[28] The remedy of emergency for cases where there even appears no hope. In accident or sudden illness, or when the patient is very frightened or terrified, or if the condition is serious enough to cause great fear to those around. If the patient is not conscious the lips may be moistened with the remedy. Other remedies in addition may also be required, as, for example, if there is unconsciousness, which is a deep, sleepy state, Clematis; if there is torture, Agrimony, and so on.

… when the fear is very great, amounting to terror or panic: either in the patient or because the condition is so serious as to cause intense fear to those around. It may be in case of sudden illness, or accident, but always when there is great emergency or danger, give the Remedy for this: made from a small plant which is called ROCK ROSE.'

Description from *The Story of the Travellers* (1934): Indication: 'Rock Rose became full of terror and was in a state of panic.' Positive outcome: 'Rock Rose in the darkest moments is just a picture of calm, serene courage.'

Group of remedies: for fear

Key words for recognising the remedy: panic, terror, nightmare

---

[28] This first sentence was omitted from most later editions of Dr. Bach's book. If refers to the 'crisis mix' that was later prepared and described by Dr. Bach.

Common expressions: 'I am panicking', 'I'm in a panic', 'I'm panically afraid.'

State of mind: this flower remedy is used only for states of mind that are urgent and disturbing and do not represent the type of the person in question. The person possibly has a terrified facial expression, pale face, palpitations, a tremor that affects their arms and legs, and their palms are sweating. A person panics because of a sudden situation or circumstance that is disturbing, not because the person is scaremonger.

Examples of situations where we might consider this remedy: any state of panic or panic fear.

Examples of people who might need this flower remedy: people who are in panic when they need to fly on a plane, or ride in an elevator, or go through a tunnel.

Positive outcome of the application of this flower remedy: sobriety in moments of great anxiety, panic and terror, quick calming in moments of panic and fear.

Examples from practice

One client contacted me after she was told during a thyroid ultrasound examination that there was an indication that the nodule on her thyroid gland was worrisome and she was consequently sent to undergo further examinations. The client was in a state of panic and said that her heart was pounding and she was out of breath at the thought of having to undergo a new examination. She was panically afraid of the puncture procedure and of what it might show. For several days she took Rock Rose flower remedy, along with Star of Bethlehem flower remedy for the shock caused by the bad news. On the day of the examination, she underwent the examination normally and did not panic, and the result was ultimately good.

Another example is one of a young woman in her early thirties, who suffered from panic attacks, and whenever she was caught up in one, she would immediately call her husband to come home from work, who then walked with her around the building in the fresh air until she calmed down. She explained that she was afraid to stay alone in the house, as she might have a heart attack, and if there was no one at home, she might die without anyone being there to help her. Her hands would start trembling from panic, her heart would be racing, so she would be even more afraid that she might have a heart attack and die.

With fear of disease and fear of heart attack, as in this case, where a client talks about a known fear – a fear we can name – this might sound like Mimulus. But when you see a case like this, which is actually an extreme version of a Mimulus state, where such known fear would produce symptoms like trembling of hands and heart pounding, this is an indication of Rock Rose – a remedy for panic fear.

If she had talked, for example, about being afraid to be left alone at home, but not knowing what she was actually afraid of at the time, then this would indicate an unknown fear and it would be a state of Aspen fear. But even then, if that unknown fear grew into an extreme state of panic, we would choose Rock Rose instead of Aspen.

We would not have chosen Rock Rose if she had said that she was afraid of a heart attack, but that she could normally stay home alone and she would not get into a state of panic when her husband was at work. Then it would be enough for her to take only Mimulus.

But because, in her case, this was a panic fear, in the period that followed she took Rock Rose flower remedy and whenever signs of panic began to appear, she would immediately take the flower remedy and that calmed her down without having to call her husband for help. After several months of regular application of Bach flower remedies, the panic attacks disappeared.

 Remember: Rock Rose flower remedy helps us to stay calm and collected in moments of panic and great fear, so that we can solve the situation in the best way possible, and react correctly and intuitively.

ROCK WATER
Spring water

Dr. Bach's description of water: 'It has long been known that certain wells and spring waters have had the power to heal some people, and such wells or springs have become renowned for this property. Any well or any spring which has been known to have had healing power and which is still left free in its natural state, unhampered by the shrines of man, may be used.'

Dr. Bach's final description of the flower remedy: 'Those who are very strict in their way of living; they deny themselves many of the joys and pleasures of life because they consider it might interfere with their work. They are hard masters to themselves. They wish to be well and strong and active, and will do anything which they believe will keep them so. They hope to be examples which will appeal to others who may then follow their ideas and be better as a result.'

Group of remedies: for over-care for welfare of others

Key words for recognising the remedy: rigour, self-discipline, self-punishment, persistence, perseverance, stubbornness

Common expressions: 'order, work, discipline', 'a healthy mind in a healthy body'.

Personality type: a person who is the Rock Water type has the strongest self-discipline among all the types of flower remedies in the Bach system. A person is willing to work hard and strenuously to achieve their goals. They are ready to give up pleasures and rest, all with the purpose of achieving perfect results in their work or progress. This person pays attention to their diet, takes regular and active exercise, and even though this can often be really difficult for them, it gives them great satisfaction to see that the hard work has paid off, and to see the result of all this to be perfect health and appearance. She strives to be a role model to others and hopes others will follow her path. This type of remedy will never break a promise made to oneself. Once established, the rules are blindly followed until the goal is achieved and she is not ready to compromise. Rock Water has a motto: 'Order, work, discipline.'

Examples of situations where we might consider this remedy: every sternness directed towards oneself:

- rigorous diet that one does not give up even when they are weak, or feeling dizzy from too few calories
- rigorous exercise that one does not give up even when they do not feel well
- abnegation, giving up food or rest, or introduction of an even more rigorous exercise plan, if they eat a cake or if they achieve poorer results in an exam or sports competition

- not sleeping and not leaving the house when the student is preparing for an exam
- non-deviation from the diet programme (vegetarian, vegan, etc.), even when the diet does not suit them and they feel weak

Examples of people who might need this flower remedy: all those who have a strict self-imposed diet and exercise regimen and similar strict self-discipline programmes, like athletes, vegetarians, vegans, models, etc.

Positive outcome of the application of this flower remedy: the person will be more open to flexibility in a self-imposed rigorous schedule, will no longer engage in self-punishing behaviour in situations where they make mistakes or achieve worse results than expected.

Examples from practice

The client contacted me for a consultation because she felt dizziness and weakness. It turned out that she had these problems because she was on a very strict diet. When I suggested she stopped the diet, she said that she should persevere in it because the diet plan needed to be implemented to the very end in order to achieve the goal she had set for herself. She still insisted that I recommend her some homeopathy for dizziness, without interrupting the diet. But I recommended Bach's Rock Water remedy instead of homeopathy. She later informed me that, that very day, immediately after taking the first dose of Bach flower remedies, she stopped her restrictive diet and started to eat normally. The dizziness also stopped the same day, as soon as she started eating more hearty meals.

Once I had a client who practised a strict exercise regime, even though she was not a professional athlete, and she could not deviate from it at any cost. She declined friends' invitations to hang out if they would arrange the meeting at a time when she was training. She imposed upon herself to go to the gym twice a day – in the morning and in the evening – noting that this rule must never be violated, no matter what. When she told me about it, I recommended her Rock Water flower remedy. A few weeks later, when she came to me for another consultation, she told me that a couple of days before, her friend had been throwing a birthday party and that she had broken her rule for the first time and gone out to dinner with her friends instead of to the gym. She said that in some other times she would have replied to such an invitation by saying that she would come to the birthday party only after her training had finished. It was the first time she realised that she needed to be flexible in her self-imposed schedule and that nothing would happen if she skipped one training session.

 Remember: Rock Water remedy frees us from unnecessary harshness towards ourselves and give us flexibility in carrying out work, health and nutrition regimes, without self-punishment.

SCLERANTHUS
Scleranthus annuus

Dr. Bach's description of the flower: '… little green Scleranthus of the cornfields …'

Dr. Bach's final description of the flower remedy: 'Those who suffer much from being unable to decide between two things, first one seeming right then the other. They are usually quiet people, and bear their difficulty alone, as they are not inclined to discuss it with others.'

Description from *The Story of the Travellers* **(1934):** Indication: 'Scleranthus had some hope but at times he suffered so from uncertainty and indecision, first wanting to take one road and almost at once another.' Positive outcome: 'Scleranthus walks with perfect certainty ...'

Group of remedies: for uncertainty

Key words for recognising the remedy: making decisions

Common expressions: the person usually talks about their dilemmas

Personality type: indecisive people who are silent and pensive when they need to make a decision; they do not ask others for advice.

Examples of situations where we might consider this remedy: any decision-making where the person does not seek the opinion of others but tries to come to a solution and decision on their own. People who need to make quick decisions in their work, without asking anyone for advice, like doctors or therapists, will benefit greatly from this flower remedy.

Examples of people who might need this flower remedy: a person trying to decide whether to accept a new job or not, a person thinking about which car to choose to buy having to choose between two cars, thinking about whether to take a loan to buy an apartment or stay in a rented apartment, whether to give another chance to save a marriage or get a divorce, a person who is considering changing their job or is considering resignation, and in all of the above situations the person does not share their dilemmas with others.

Positive outcome of the application of this flower remedy: the person will easily make the decision that is right, will feel relieved.

Examples from practice

I once had a client who came to me for help. She was several weeks pregnant and was tormented by a great dilemma, which she could not share with anyone. Namely, she was afraid that the child would be too much of a responsibility for her because she already had two small children and confided in me that she had a abortion scheduled for the next day. But she was still worried about that decision and she wasn't sure she was doing the right thing. I recommended her to take Scleranthus flower remedy, as often as possible during the day, so that she could know what was best for her by the next morning. She called me several days later and said she had decided to keep the baby. She did not go to the scheduled appointment for the abortion. She gave birth to a child and sent me a touching thank you note after his birth. It was one of the most special cases in my practice. That client still calls me today and regularly sends me pictures of her child.

Another example was a client who had marital problems and was considering initiating divorce proceedings. She wanted to stay with her husband for the sake of her son, and yet again, she was not sure if anything could be fixed in their relationship, even if she stayed married. After talking to her, I recommended her Scleranthus flower remedy for the decision she needed to make and about which she hadn't told anyone, as well as Holly for the anger she felt towards her husband. After one bottle of flower remedy, she sent me a message in which she described how much love for her husband she felt again, 'like fire', and that she had decided to stay with him. She soon became pregnant and gave birth to another child. Scleranthus was the flower remedy that showed her so very quickly and easily what was the best decision for her. You can read the impressions of that client in the example for Holly flower remedy.

> *Remember: Scleranthus helps us make decisions that we normally cannot share with others. This flower remedy will help us find the best solution faster and easier, instead of struggling day and night with thinking about a possible outcome.*

STAR OF BETHLEHEM
Ornithogalum umbellatum

Dr. Bach's final description of the flower remedy: 'For those in great distress under conditions which for a time produce great unhappiness. The shock of serious news, the loss of some one[29] dear, the fright following an accident, and such like. For those who for a time refuse to be consoled[30] this remedy brings comfort.'

Group of remedies: for despondency or despair

Key words for recognising the remedy: shock, bad news

Common expressions: 'I'm in shock.'

---

[29]   In later editions 'some one' is usually written as 'someone'. The Bach Centre preferred to leave 'some one', to be in line with Dr. Bach's other texts.

[30]   Most later editions of dr. Bach's book insert a comma after 'consoled'.

State of mind: this flower remedy does not represent the type of person, but is applied only in situations of great stress and shock that a person suddenly experiences; the person might be shaking and confused.

Examples of situations where we might consider this remedy: accident, misfortune, bad news.

Examples of people who might need this flower remedy: all persons who have experienced shock due to some of the following or similar situations:

- news of a poor medical finding
- news of a person's death
- news of an accident or mishap
- resignation
- sudden termination of a love affair
- robbery
- turbulence in an aircraft
- sudden surgery
- sudden termination of pregnancy
- all other situations that present great stress and shock to the person

Positive outcome of the application of this flower remedy: the person will calm down and the shock will not leave negative consequences on the mind and body.

Note: by applying this flower remedy it is possible to cleanse both the old traumas and shocks that a person has experienced, no matter how long ago these occurred. If a person still suffers from the negative consequences of some stress and shock, this flower remedy will be extremely good for them and will enable them to finally get over the event.

Examples from practice

I often give this flower remedy to clients who come to me for consultations after having received some bad news, most often a diagnosis of a disease they have unexpectedly received. For example, I recently had a consultation with a young woman who was diagnosed with CIN 3 and was about to undergo a Letz procedure at the hospital. The same week, she received two diagnoses – CIN 3 and a recommendation to remove the complete thyroid gland. In shock and disbelief, she came to me, seeking solace for her condition. The Star of Bethlehem flower remedy calmed her down that same day and she was able to look at her situation more calmly. She continued to take this flower remedy and calmly performed the Letz procedure, which went painlessly and smoothly. She sought another opinion for the thyroid, and didn't need surgery after all.

Another client called me after a minor collision she had experienced while driving to work. An ambulance took her to the hospital for an examination just to make sure she was alright and to determine her condition. She told me that she was in shock after the crash, that she was pale and that she was beside herself. Luckily, she had a bottle of crisis mix in her purse, so she was taking this all the way to the hospital. The doctors determined that she was fine, and she calmed down very quickly after the initial shock. Fortunately, the remedy Star of Bethlehem, which is an integral part of crisis mix, had an effect and calmed her down very quickly. The condition she described was a typical description of the Star of Bethlehem flower remedy.

Important note: this flower remedy is not a substitute for emergency medical and professional help!

 Remember: Star of Bethlehem flower remedy helps us keep our composure and peace in situations of great shock.

SWEET CHESTNUT
Castanea vulgaris[31]

Dr. Bach's final description of the flower remedy: 'For those moments which happen to some people when the anguish is so great as to seem to be unbearable. When the mind or body feels as if it had borne to the uttermost limit of its endurance, and that now it must give way. When it seems there is nothing but destruction and annihilation left to face.'

Group of remedies: for despondency or despair

Key words for recognising the remedy: unbearable mental suffering, 'dark night of the soul'.

Common expressions: 'this is unbearable', 'I can feel my strength ebbing away', 'I won't be able to stand this any more.'

State of mind: this flower remedy does not represent the type of person, but the person finds themselves in a situation where mental suffering is unbearable and they feel they have reached the limit of their endurance.

---

[31] Modern name: *Castanea sativa*.

Examples of situations where we might consider this remedy:

- 'soul pain' after the loss of a loved one
- a difficult life situation that is unbearable and seems like the 'end of the world'

Examples of people who might need this flower remedy: those who have reached the limit of their endurance due to the mental suffering they are experiencing.

Positive outcome of the application of this flower remedy: the person feels relief and develops new hope that the situation will improve. They get the strength to endure. They get an insight into why suffering was a necessity. They look at the situation from a positive angle.

Examples from practice

A client who was a single mother and in a difficult life situation called me and said that her situation had become too difficult for her and that the emotional pain she was feeling was unbearable. Since she already knew how to use Bach flower remedies on her own – because she had previously attended education about them – I reminded her that she should take Sweet Chestnut for this condition. She took it in frequent doses throughout the evening, and after the first dose she calmed down and felt positive.

On one occasion, a person in a very serious emotional condition came to me for a consultation after the tragic loss of a loved one. She told me she was torn by an unbearable emotional pain in her heart and soul. She could not find consolation in anything. I also put Sweet Chestnut in her personal mix, which matched the sentences she uttered. After the first bottle, she was already in a better condition, and through long-term consultations over the course of a year, she managed to solve all the emotional problems that were associated with this great trauma.

> *Remember: Sweet Chestnut flower remedy will free us from a state of agony and despair, when it seems impossible to move on, and when emotional suffering and pain are too great and unbearable. This flower remedy will show us a ray of light in the darkness, and give us new meaning and hope to persevere and endure.*

VERVAIN
Verbena officinalis

Dr. Bach's description of the flower: 'Vervain, the little mauve flower of the hedge-banks …'

Dr. Bach's final description of the flower remedy: 'Those with fixed principles and ideas, which they are confident are right, and which they very rarely change. They have a great wish to convert all around them to their own views of life. They are strong of will and have much courage when they are convinced of those things that they wish to teach. In illness they struggle on long after many would have given up their duties.'

Description from *The Story of the Travellers* **(1934):** Indication: 'Vervain should also have known the path well enough, but although he had become a little confused, held forth at length as to the only way out of the wood.' Positive outcome: 'Vervain no longer preaches but silently points the way.'

Group of remedies: for over-care for welfare of others

Key words for recognising the remedy: activist

Common expressions: 'Try it, it will help you!', 'This is phenomenal, you have to try it!'

Personality type: activist, justice fighter. The person tries to convert the people around them to the lifestyle and methods they practise and which they consider to be the best and the only correct ones. Talks in enthusiastic manner of speech, and has a positive life attitude.

Examples of situations where we might consider this remedy: losing a sense of perspective because of passionately held beliefs; over-enthusiasm.

Examples of people who might need this flower remedy: anybody with a strong sense of principle who finds it hard to control their passion, such as:

- vegetarians and vegans in the company of meat eaters
- non-smoker in the company of smokers
- a homeopath or Bach practitioner in the company of people who do not believe in homeopathy and Bach flower remedies
- a religious fanatic who seeks to convert others to their faith
- an activist for the protection of other people's rights

Positive outcome of the application of this flower remedy: the person understands that each person has their own path, that everyone has the right to their own life choices. A person will not harass other people by persuading them to choose the lifestyle and methods they advocate and preach. A person realises that it is not always the time or place for them to 'preach', and is able to refrain and remain silent if no one has asked for their opinion.

Note: Vervain and Oak are the two remedies that have the most strength to fight in a state of illness. Those two flower remedies never give up.

Oak fights for his life to the last breath and never gives up. Oak seems to have inexhaustible physical and mental strength.

Vervain always has a positive outlook on life and until their last breath will believe that there is a cure for them, and will always actively seek for a solution to their condition or illness. Vervain has inexhaustible positive energy.

Examples from practice

A client who was a Vervain type started coming to my centre for counselling on Bach flower remedies for her dog. She was an active animal rights activist and over time began to use Bach flower remedies for herself as well, but also to learn about the remedies so she could further spread that knowledge. The change I noticed in her was visible after she had been taking Vervain flower remedy for several months and in several personal bottles. The sturdy activist in her, who wanted to convince every dog owner to take the right path — the path she saw as the only real one and that she herself practised — balanced out over time. She noticed that she was less obtrusive in her approach to other animal owners, and became aware that not every dog owner is open to treating their pet with homeopathy and Bach flower remedies. She learned to discern the appropriate moment for discussing these methods, and when it was neither the time nor the place to do so.

Another client used every seminar break, while we were having lunch together, as an opportunity to comment on our food choices, and to try to persuade us that her diet was the best, as well as to instruct us on how we should buy groceries, cook and eat the way she eats. Other seminar participants also agreed that her type was Vervain, so during the seminar and the exercises we did at the seminar, jokingly drew her attention to the fact that Vervain was her type and that it would be good for her to start using this flower remedy. While I have no feedback on whether she took this flower remedy and what progress she has made, this is a typical example of the Vervain type of person, who tries to convert everyone around them to their lifestyle and convince them of their core life beliefs.

I myself went through a Vervain phase, when I tried to direct everyone around me to try Bach flower remedies, convinced that it was the solution to all of the problems in the world and for all of the people in the world. I literally used to mix flower remedies together for people who did not ask me to do it and who were not interested in my enthusiasm for the remedies. After using Vervain flower remedy, I achieved balance. Today I talk about the methods I practise only if someone asks me for help, if they ask me to explain to them how these methods work, and if they are interested. Today I teach about these remedies and I am happy to be able to express thereby my Vervain type, knowing that the people I teach have signed up for the seminar themselves and that they want to learn about the remedies. I have learned to recognise the place and time when it is appropriate to talk about the methods in which I believe so deeply and which I practise.

> *Remember: Vervain flower remedy teaches us to respect other people's choices and other people's paths of development, without having the need to convert others to our path. With this flower remedy we realise that everyone has their own pace of development, their own path and their own freedom of choice, without feeling dissatisfaction and disappointment because they do not practise the same things as ourselves.*

VINE

Vitis vinifera

Dr. Bach's final description of the flower remedy: 'Very capable people, certain of their own ability, confident of success. Being so assured, they think that it would be for the benefit of others if they could be persuaded to do things as they themselves do, or as they are certain is right. Even in illness they will direct their attendants. They may be of great value in emergency.'

Group of remedies: for over-care for welfare of others

Key words for recognising the remedy: dictator, leader

Common expressions: 'Do as I say!', 'That's the way it is, full stop!', 'It is non-negotiable!'

Personality type: a person who has a dominant, strong and intimidating attitude. They even have a threatening and aggressive attitude. They often shout and issue orders. Director of a company. The head of a family. Boss at work. President. Leader. A dominant partner who demands obedience. A dominant parent that children fear. Aggressive person.

Examples of situations where we might consider this remedy: all situations in which the above types of persons find themselves, when they restrict other people's free will, when they intimidate and harass others.

Examples of people who might need this flower remedy: see personality type.

Positive outcome of the application of this flower remedy: the person is ready to negotiate and compromise. The person is ready to hear what the other party has to say and how the other party feels. They understand the suffering and pain they cause in another person. They realise that maybe what they think is best for the other person may actually not be the best, and they see alternatives and compromise solutions.

Examples from practice

My clients often complain about the Vine person in their life. It is usually a dominant person who may be a director, a parent, a partner, a spouse, who controls their life and actions by issuing orders and by taking a strict dominant approach.

The problem is how to point out to a Vine person that they are harassing us and how to give them the remedies?

The trick is to focus on strengthening your own personality, not on changing others. Thus a person who has a Vine dictator and tyrant in their life should take Centaury flower remedy, in order to empower themselves and to stand up for themselves (see the examples written under Centaury flower remedy).

Vine will rarely come to consultations and ask for remedies for themselves because they have realised that they are harassing other people. However, I was lucky that on one occasion a client came to me with such a story.

It was a retired lady whose husband had died, and she lived in the same house as her children, their spouses and her grandchildren. So, three generations of family under one roof. The lady very charmingly presented that she is the head of the family and that her task is to align each of them. She noticed everything that each family member was doing wrong and gave them clear instructions on what they should do. She literally told me that she was driving them crazy, but that she had to treat them that way because she knew what was best for them and that they were not able to see it for themselves. So, during the first consultation she told me: 'I have just come to see how you do it, and now that I see that you are doing it well, I will send them all to you to put them in order.' And that's how it was. Soon, they were all coming to me one by one for consultations. Often the lady would try to tell me how to deal with them and what therapies to recommend or what problems to solve. A real example of a Vine person! We were all supposed to obey her orders. I, of course, worked with each of them according to their needs and in the manner they asked me to, regardless of the instructions I received from Vine, the head of the family. With their stories they also confirmed that the mother dominates their lives and they often described situations from their daily lives and communication. Although they were a complex family in terms of counselling, I have to admit that they were very likeable and that their stories amused me in some way. I loved working with them because I always heard stories from all angles and perspectives. May I say that I liked the mother best and found her to be most charming, and that in her stories I could really recognise genuine care for her family? She was fully aware of her role and the way they all saw her and came to ask for help – both for herself and for them. I find that my work with this family truly enriched my practice.

> *Remember: Vine flower remedy teaches us to respect other people's feelings and needs, without having the need to dominate them and tell them how to live their lives. With this flower remedy we become open to compromise and begin to realise that others should have the same rights and freedom of action as we have.*

WALNUT
Juglans regia

Dr. Bach's final description of the flower remedy: 'For those who have definite ideals and ambitions in life and are fulfilling them, but on rare occasions are tempted to be led away from their own ideas, aims and work by the enthusiasm, convictions or strong opinions of others. The remedy gives constancy and protection from outside influences.'

Group of remedies: for those over-sensitive to influences and ideas

Key words for recognising the remedy: change, protection from negative influences

Common expressions: 'I don't seem to be able to adjust', 'I feel bad after talking to these people', 'these people drain all my energy', 'I absorb all that.'

State of mind or personality type: a person who is sometimes tempted to be led away from their aims. A person who finds it difficult to get used to new circumstances. A person who is sensitive to other people's energies and emotions, and 'takes everything to heart'. A state of exhaustion and mood swings after spending time with other people.

Examples of situations where we might consider this remedy:

- all periods of life transition – starting kindergarten and school, pregnancy, childbirth, birth of a new child, moving to a new apartment or another country, changing jobs, retirement, puberty, menopause, marriage, divorce, etc., if a person finds it difficult to get used to these new circumstances

- exposure to negative people, if the person feels they need protection from these negative energies

- adaptation to sleeping in a hotel, on the road; adaptation to ride on a boat, in a car or plane, if a person finds it difficult to get used to these new circumstances

- staying in an environment where people eat, drink or smoke, and the person has decided to start a restrictive diet, not to drink alcohol or not to smoke, and feels they might be tempted to be led away from their goals

Examples of people who might need this flower remedy: a person who works with people, especially in workplaces where people wait in line and where negative energies are generated – for example, in a hospital, in a shop, in a bank, in a post office, etc. – and when a person believes they need protection from these negative energies. Therapists and doctors who work with people who are sick, depressed, angry, impatient, frightened, etc., and when a person believes they need protection from these negative energies.

Positive outcome of the application of this flower remedy:

• protection from external negative influences and people

• perseverance in a decision, not allowing other people to tempt us to break the decision made

• adaptation to new circumstances in periods of transition

Note: Walnut flower remedy will help a person persevere in their decision, but only if the person has already made a decision. This remedy cannot be given to a person without their knowledge in order to resist alcohol, alcoholic beverages or cigarettes without the person having themselves voluntarily made the decision to refrain from consuming said substances.

'The Walnut Tree', story by Dr. Bach (1935)

'This remedy, Walnut, is the remedy of advancing stages: teething, puberty, change of life.

Also for the big decisions made during life, such as change of religion, change of occupation, change of country.

It is the remedy for a great change. The remedy for those who have decided to take a great step forward in life. The decision to step forward, to break old conventions, to leave old limits and restrictions, and to start on a new and better way, often brings with it physical suffering because of the slight regrets, the slight heart-breakings at severance from old ties, old associations, old thoughts.

This remedy will soothe and help to abolish the physical reactions under such conditions, whether the step forward being taken is of a mental or physical nature.

It is the remedy which helps us to pass through all such states without regrets, without memories of the past, without fears for the future, and therefore saves us from the mental and physical suffering which is so often associated with such events.

Undoubtedly a great spell-breaker, both of things of the past commonly called heredity, and circumstances of the present.'

Examples from practice

This is the remedy that I adore and I often recommend. Since it provides protection from external influences, my employees and I regularly take this flower remedy so that we can work with people without hindrance. Our clients can be sad, unhappy, angry, nervous, impatient or depressed, and none of that is transferred to us, so we manage to professionally converse with all our clients.

Therefore, I recommend this flower remedy to clients who works with people, and who are very much affected by other people's negative emotions. These are especially people who work with seriously ill people or sick children, and they often ask me for the remedy to help them and to give them protection from these negative emotions.

Some of my clients, who are lawyers, school teachers, speech therapists, nurses and even judges, regularly use this flower remedy when working with people. Clients who work as waiters, ambulance drivers, lawyers, managers also say that Walnut flower remedy helps them as protection from the negative influences of others.

And I recommend them to facilitate adaptation, when this is needed, since all my clients at some point go through some stages of adaptation. Also to clients who have decided to go on a diet, so they can stick to their decisions.

> *Remember: Walnut flower remedy provides us with protection from negative people and situations, keeps us from deviating from the path we have chosen, because of others, and makes it easier for us to adapt to new situations.*

WATER VIOLET
Hottonia palustris

Dr. Bach's description of the flower: '… beautiful Water Violet, which floats so freely on the surface of our clearest streams …'

Dr. Bach's final description of the flower remedy: 'For those who in health or illness like to be alone. Very quiet people, who move about without noise, speak little, and then gently. Very independent, capable and self-reliant. Almost free of the opinions of others. They are aloof, leave people alone and go their own way. Often clever and talented. Their peace and calmness is a blessing to those around them.'

Description from *The Story of the Travellers* **(1934):** Indication: 'Water Violet had travelled that way before and knew the right road and yet was a little proud and a little disdainful that others did not understand. Water Violet thought them a little inferior.'[32] Positive outcome: '… Water Violet, more like an angel than a man, passes amongst the company like a breath of warm wind or a ray of glorious sunshine, blessing everyone.'

Group of remedies: for loneliness

Key words for recognising the remedy: self-confidence, isolation, loneliness

Some mistaken perceptions people might have of Water Violet people are arrogance, haughtiness, conceit, but they aren't really how it feels to be a Water Violet person. Have these in mind, though, as you may get this impression of a Water Violet person, or you may hear from a Water Violet that people see them this way.

Common expressions: 'I like being alone', 'I like it best when I'm alone.'

Personality type: a self-confident person, aware of their knowledge and qualities, who loves solitude or the company of only a few close friends. Others see them as an inaccessible and conceited person, a loner. This type of person has no problems with self-confidence. They have a dignified attitude. Sometimes they do not talk much when in company but rather just observe others.

Examples of situations where we might consider this remedy: all situations where a person feels lonely, even though

---

[32]   See Dr. Bach's final description of Water Violet above, where he described Water Violet as self-reliant and independent. He did not use the words pride and disdain in the final description. See page 23 of www.bachcentre.com/wp-content/uploads/2019/10/Twelve_Healers_1941.pdf, The Bach Centre (2019).

they are the ones who have chosen to isolate themselves.

Examples of people who might need this flower remedy: all those who love to isolate from others in their privacy, but eventually feel lonely.

Positive outcome of the application of this flower remedy: after applying this flower remedy, the person will not feel lonely any more. They will start to open up to more people, not just their few close friends, when they have a need to socialise with others.

Examples from practice

During the periods of movement restriction required in 2020–21 due to the Covid-19 pandemic, I identified several typical examples of people who are of the Water Violet type.

A Water Violet person by nature likes to be alone and often prefers to practise quiet activities such as reading a book or walking independently in nature. These are people who enjoy sitting alone in peace and quiet, or spending peaceful moments socialising with a few close friends. In the course of the pandemic, I was explicitly able to identify Water Violet individuals by their reaction to self-isolation or restriction of movement.

Water Violet people have regularly told me that it is not at all difficult for them to spend time at home in self-isolation because it is something they do anyway, under normal circumstances. They didn't miss hanging out in cafés, the noise and crowds of people. They really enjoyed these peaceful moments at home.

However, I didn't automatically recommend Water Violet flower remedy to such people just because they like to spend time alone. The remedy is needed only in those situations where people start to feel lonely. So, for example, it was needed by a client who usually likes to spend time alone, but had begun to feel lonely and said she would like to have more opportunities to socialise with friends. She even missed dinners out with a large number of acquaintances and associates, events she had previously hated and avoided. After taking Water Violet, she no longer felt lonely and says now that she feels ready for more socialising, with a wider circle of friends, when the pandemic ends.

An example of the opposite of this remedy is the Agrimony type, who loves to socialise with a large number of people and is generally a very sociable person. My experience of clients of the Agrimony type was that they found it particularly difficult to bear the restrictions on movement and assembly, and the ban on the operation of cafés and restaurants during the pandemic. For them, staying in the house, in silence and solitude, was a real punishment.

> *Remember:* Water Violet remedy help us to banish feelings of loneliness in situations we have created ourselves by withdrawing into isolation. It helps us to open up more easily to outings and other people when we need to do so, so that we can share our peace and composure with others. With this remedy we can more easily achieve a balance between socialising and the moments of solitude, peace and quiet that we love.

WHITE CHESTNUT

Aesculus hippocastanum

White Chestnut is so named to enable us to distinguish it from the bud of the same tree, which is used to prepare the flower remedy of Chestnut Bud. (See the section on the boiling method earlier in the book.)

Dr. Bach's final description of the flower remedy: 'For those who cannot prevent thoughts, ideas, arguments which they do not desire from entering their minds. Usually at such times when the interest of the moment is not strong enough to keep the mind full. Thoughts which worry and will remain, or if for a time thrown out, will return. They seem to circle round and round and cause mental torture. The presence of such unpleasant thoughts drives out peace and interferes with being able to think only of the work or pleasure of the day.'

Group of remedies: for insufficient interest in present circumstances

Key words for recognising the remedy: mental anguish, unwanted thoughts, negative thoughts, disturbing thoughts, lack of concentration, insomnia due to unwanted thoughts

Common expressions: 'those negative thoughts haunt me', 'I cannot stop those negative thoughts', 'those thoughts go through my head non-stop', 'I cannot fall asleep from those thoughts', 'those thoughts don't allow me to concentrate'.

State of mind: a person who ruminates over negative experiences, a person who talks internally to people who hurt them, goes over and over through scenarios that happened earlier, are worried, do not listen to what is being said to them because they are thinking about something else that bothers them.

Examples of situations where we might consider this remedy: for people who cannot fall asleep due to unwanted thoughts, during exams when a person is bothered by sounds in the classroom.

Examples of people who might need this flower remedy: students and pupils when studying, lecturers during lectures, performers during performances, people suffering from insomnia before sleeping (if insomnia is caused by unwanted thoughts).

Positive outcome of the application of this flower remedy: the person doesn't have any more disturbing, unwanted thoughts.

The difference between White Chestnut and Red Chestnut: 'The presence of those unpleasant thoughts prevents peace and does not allow a person to think only about their daily obligations or about pleasures.'

A common feature – the inability to independently turn off unwanted thoughts.

Red Chestnut – cannot relax on a business trip or on a romantic trip with a partner because they worry about the children left at home. A person is constantly thinking about the children, and cannot indulge in enjoyment or concentrate on work.

White Chestnut – cannot relax on vacation because they are thinking about problems at work. They cannot fall asleep because they keep reiterating in their head conversations they had earlier that day, or imagining a possible conversation scenario they are going to have the next day, and they cannot voluntarily dismiss those thoughts.

Examples from practice

This is the flower remedy that I personally use before lectures, when I need to concentrate better on what I am teaching, without being disturbed by some other thoughts or some worries that are disrupting my flow of thoughts. Also, if I need to concentrate on writing a book or learning a subject, this is the flower remedy that always keeps my concentration at a very high level. This was also the first Bach flower remedy that I took, at a time when I needed it most, for insomnia while writing my master's thesis.

Here are the impressions of one of my clients who used this Bach flower remedy during her studies and exams in college. I have underlined the parts of the text that accurately describe the effects of the White Chestnut remedy so that we can clearly discern them and remember their action.

'I had my first experience with Bach flower remedies before a very important exam at the university. After three days of using Bach flower remedies, my concentration increased, a desire to learn suddenly appeared and, what's more, I was very calm, composed and concentrated on what I was doing. On the day of the exam I put my flower remedies in a bottle of water that was constantly by my side. Sipping water during the exam, the flower remedy calmed me down and I was focused only on the paper in front of me. No external stimuli prevented me from writing the exam, neither colleagues who were fidgeting nor the traffic and street noise. In addition, I had never before experienced such calmness and concentration during an important exam, without traces of panic or concern about whether or not I would know an answer, and whether I would complete the exam on time.

I would describe the effect of Bach flower remedies as similar to the feeling of being placed in a protective capsule, in which you are concentrating only on yourself and nothing can distract or disturb you.'

> *Remember: White Chestnut flower remedy ensures focus and drives away unwanted thoughts that disturb us and interfere with our normal functioning, sleep and thinking. This flower remedy gives us the power of positive thinking when we need to get rid of disruptive thoughts.*

WILD OAT
Bromus asper[33]

Dr. Bach's final description of the flower remedy: 'Those who have ambitions to do something of prominence in life, who wish to have much experience, and to enjoy all that which is possible for them, to take life to the full. Their difficulty is to determine what occupation to follow; as although their ambitions are strong, they have no calling which appeals to them above all others. This may cause delay and dissatisfaction.'

Group of remedies: for uncertainty

Key words for recognising the remedy: decision making, turning point in life, choosing a life path, finding a life purpose and vocation

Common expressions: 'I'm at a turning point in my life', 'I'm at a crossroad and I don't know which way to go.'

---

[33] Modern name: *Bromus ramosus.*

State of mind or personality type: a person who has difficulty finding their life purpose and their life path. They are constantly looking for something to fulfil them, and they do not know what that would be.

Examples of situations where we might consider this remedy: making a life decision.

Examples of people who might need this flower remedy: a child who is about to choose a high school or college, a person who is about to decide on the job they will be doing, the country they are going to live in or their life partner – if they are at a crossroads and need help to choose their life path.

Positive outcome of the application of this flower remedy: the person discovers their path, the one that is best for them. They make a decision with ease and with certainty that it is the right choice for them. They believe that the direction they have chosen is for their highest good.

Examples from practice

One of my clients, who attended my seminars and learned some of the methods I practise myself, was discouraged about choosing her life path. She didn't know which path to take and what she should do next in life. She was unemployed at the time she came to see me. I recommended Wild Oat flower remedy to her, and after a few weeks she called me completely thrilled. She had decided to start her own business, for which she even received incentives from the state, and she enrolled in further courses and training in order to improve her knowledge. The flower remedy provided an answer to her doubts related to the choice of her life direction. Today she successfully runs her own business.

I can confirm the positive outcome of the application of this flower remedy because this is the one that opened my eyes and showed me my life path. The result of Wild Oat's action was that I embarked on the road of homeopathy and opened my own homeopathic centre.

I also gave this flower remedy to my older daughter, Helena, when she needed to choose her direction and submit her papers for high school enrolment. She was taking Wild Oat for several weeks before the enrolment period. Although she had been talking about enrolling in one of the gymnasium high schools for months and had good grades, in the end she changed her mind at the last minute and decided to enrol in the school of economics. She chose the school completely on her own, without the influence and interference of others, and I made certain that she would do that by adding Walnut flower remedy to the same bottle. My husband and I allowed her to decide for herself about choosing a school, and the flower remedies helped her see all the pros and cons of each school and to easily make a decision.

 Remember: Wild Oat is a flower remedy that helps us find our life vocation, choose the right path when we are at a turning point in life, and boldly step towards fulfilling our goals and desires.

WILD ROSE
Rosa canina

Dr. Bach's final description of the flower remedy: 'Those who without apparently sufficient reason become resigned to all that happens, and just glide through life, take it as it is, without any effort to improve things and find some joy. They have surrendered to the struggle of life without complaint.'

Group of remedies: for insufficient interest in present circumstances

Key words for recognising the remedy: listlessness, apathy, giving in to destiny and situation

Common expressions: 'That's life', 'It is what it is', 'Nothing can be done about it', 'That cannot be changed', 'It is impossible to change that.'

Personality type: a listless, apathetic person who is not happy with their life, job, partner, etc., but does nothing to change that. The person has simply acquiesced to life as it is.

Examples of situations where we might consider this remedy: any dissatisfaction with one's life situation.

Examples of people who might need this flower remedy: a person who has no hobbies, is not satisfied with their job, has no motivation or realisation that it is possible to change something in life.

Positive outcome of the application of this flower remedy: the person realises that the power is in their hands and that it is possible to make some changes in life. They start making decisions, enrol in courses on desired hobbies, they change jobs or start looking for a new job.

The difference between Wild Rose and Hornbeam: both remedies encourage a person to be active and motivate them to get moving. Hornbeam helps a person who feels mentally and physically tired even at the thought of a task to be done, and does not have the strength to make themselves move and tackle the task at hand. Wild Rose thinks it is impossible to change the circumstances that make them feel dissatisfied, so they do not even realise that something can change and that something should be done. Wild Rose is unaware that they can do something to feel better and more fulfilled in life.

Hornbeam – *a task* they <u>know</u> they have to complete, but have no strength to do so.

Wild Rose – *life circumstances* with which they are not satisfied, but <u>do not realise</u> that they can actually do something to change them.

Examples from practice

I have so far recommended Wild Rose several times in my practice, to people who have acquiesced to life without trying to change or initiate anything. For example, I had a client who was extremely unhappy at work and always complained about being stuck in that situation and position. She did not see any possibility of that changing. She was taking Wild Rose flower remedy, and began to consider other options and other jobs. Very quickly she got an offer to move to another company with much better working conditions.

Another client was unemployed and did not see any possibility of finding employment. She took a bottle of Wild Rose and called me the following week to tell me that she had decided to start her own business.

The third example is a client who was fired and spent months sitting at home depressed, without direction or any orientation regarding what she should do. She came to me for a consultation in a listless state typical of Wild Rose. After one bottle of Wild Rose flower remedy, she applied for a job at a company and was hired immediately.

Remember: Wild Rose gives us a new impetus, strength and will to change those things and circumstances in life that make us unhappy.

WILLOW

Salix vitellina

Dr. Bach's final description of the flower remedy: 'For those who have suffered adversity or misfortune and find these difficult to accept, without complaint or resentment, as they judge life much by the success which it brings. They feel that they have not deserved so great a trial, that it was unjust, and they become embittered. They often take less interest and less activity[34] in those things of life which they had previously enjoyed.'

Group of remedies: for despondency or despair

Key words for recognising the remedy: bitterness, resentment, self-pity, blaming others

Common expressions: 'poor me', 'they did it to me', 'they are to blame', 'no one loves me', 'everyone has that except me'.

State of mind or personality type: a person who could be the Willow type considers themselves a victim, is resentful of those who have hurt them, feels that they have been unfairly deprived of something or hurt.

Examples of situations where we might consider this remedy: situation where a person feels they have been unfairly deprived of something or hurt.

---

[34] Text written in later editions of Dr. Bach's book: 'They often take less interest and are less active …'.

Examples of people who might need this flower remedy: a bitter person, a person who feels sorry for themself, a person who feels they are a victim of injustice.

Positive outcome of the application of this flower remedy: helps the person to understand other people, and release anger, resentment and bitterness. They are accepting of their share of guilt and responsibility in the situation.

The difference between Holly and Willow – anger:

Holly is angry and wants to get revenge and hurt the other person. He wants to see the person who hurt or angered him suffer. He thinks of revenge, he wants revenge, he wishes evil and suffering on the person he is angry at.

Willow is angry and wants the person who hurt her to realise that it was wrong and how much she is suffering because of it at the moment. She believes she has been wronged and wants an apology. She will be bitter and angry until she gets an apology and until she sees that the person has realised that he has not treated her properly. She is able to bear that grudge for years, taking the role of a victim, sufferer and martyr.

Examples from practice

At the beginning of my practice, when I first opened my centre, I worked with a client who was a real Willow type. She was divorced and even though it had been more than seven or eight years since she divorced, she still felt sorry for herself, sorry that it had happened to her, and she always used to tell that sad story, with a lot of self-pity, lamentation and lingering bitterness towards her ex-husband. The question 'Why me?' could always be explicitly heard in her stories, as well as the words 'not fair'. In addition, she felt bitterness and resentment towards her parents, who she felt had never loved her or understood her enough. And even with regards to that relationship with her parents, the language of Willow flower remedy could be heard, saying 'Poor me, no one loves me.' She blamed both her ex-husband and her parents for her problems. But gradually, after several bottles of flower remedies, she began to accept her share of responsibility in those relationships, and slowly let go of that Willow condition and behaviour. She realised what a Willow person represents and told me how she had accepted and grown to love this flower remedy. She began to learn about Bach flower remedies and to work on her personal progress. This was one of the most difficult, but also one of the most successful, cases I have had in my practice. She took many bottles of flower remedies and homeopathic remedies, but she became aware of her basic, Willow type. Even today, she sometimes calls me and thanks me because after many years she is still well and stable.

 Remember: Willow flower remedy helps us overcome sadness, anger and resentment, to get over and let go of situations in which we have been hurt by others.

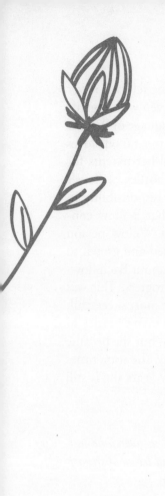

PART THREE

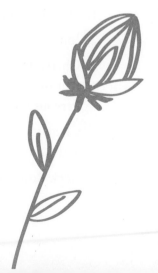

THE CRISIS MIX FORMULA

Dr. Bach devised this combination for crisis situations, when he realised that during emergencies there is no time to mix flower remedies, that it is necessary to have ready-made flower remedies, in a bag or in a pocket, that can be used immediately to calm the person and help them overcome shock or crisis.

The composition of the crisis mix remedy is as follows:

1. Star of Bethlehem – shock, stress, bad news, trauma

2. Impatiens – irritability, haste in stressful situations

3. Cherry Plum – a person feeling that they will go crazy, that they cannot cope with a situation, on the verge of a nervous breakdown, uncontrolled violent reactions

4. Clematis – feeling of fainting and weakness due to shock and panic

5. Rock Rose – panic, dread and danger

CRISIS MIX CREAM

Crisis mix cream was designed and made by Dr. Bach's collaborator Nora Weeks.

The composition of crisis mix cream is as follows:

1. Star of Bethlehem – shock, stress, bad news, trauma

2. Impatiens – irritability, haste in stressful situations

3. Cherry Plum – a person feeling that they will go crazy, that they cannot cope with a situation, on the verge of a nervous breakdown, uncontrolled violent reactions

4. Clematis – the person feels that they will lose consciousness

5. Rock Rose – panic and dread

6. Crab Apple – feeling sick, dirty

Tip: for beauty and freshness of the skin, use Bach's crisis mix cream as a day or night cream. In the morning, the cream will prepare you for a stress-free day, and in the evening it will relax you and help you unwind before you go to bed.

Personally, I am a big supporter of using Bach crisis mix cream as a day and night face cream, and all my clients with whom I sometimes discuss beauty tips know this. Both I and my family members have been using this cream as a face cream for many years.

I have also received feedback from clients about the benefits of using this cream. One even boasted that her hairdresser asked her, after several months of consecutive use of the cream, if she'd had a facelift.

METHODS OF DOSAGE

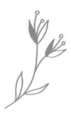

Dr. Edward Bach gave clear instructions[35] for dosage in his book *The Twelve Healers and Other Remedies*:

'As all these remedies are pure and harmless, there is no fear of giving too much or too often, though only the smallest quantities are necessary to act as a dose. Nor can any remedy do harm should it prove not to be the one actually needed for the case.

To prepare, take about two drops from the stock bottle into a small bottle nearly filled with water; if this is required to keep for some time a little brandy may be added as a preservative.

This bottle is used for giving doses, and but a few drops of this, taken in a little water, milk, or any way convenient, is all that is necessary.

In urgent cases the doses may be given every few minutes, until there is improvement; in severe cases about half-hour-

---

[35] The dosage instructions were rewritten in later editions of *The Twelve Healers*. See pages 23 and 24 of www.bachcentre.com/wp-content/uploads/2019/10/Twelve_Healers_1941.pdf, The Bach Centre (2019).

ly; and in long-standing cases every two or three hours, or more often or less as the patient feels the need.

In those unconscious, moisten the lips frequently.

Whenever there is pain, stiffness, inflammation, or any local trouble, in addition a lotion should be applied. Take a few drops from the medicine bottle in a bowl of water and in this soak a piece of cloth and cover the affected part; this can be kept moist from time to time, as necessary.

Sponging or bathing in water with a few drops of the remedies added may at times be useful.'

FREQUENTLY ASKED QUESTIONS

How is my personal bottle of Bach flower remedies prepared?

Your personal bottle is prepared by taking two drops of each of the remedies you need and placing them in a glass bottle using a 30 ml pipette. If the crisis mix remedy is added to a personal bottle, even though it is a mixture of five remedies it is counted as one remedy in this case (for stress) and four drops are used because it contains a smaller amount of each of the individual parent tinctures from which it has been prepared. Then the bottle is filled almost to the top with water and a teaspoon of brandy is added as a preservative.

If you are sensitive to alcohol or for some other reason do not wish to or cannot consume products that contain alcohol, non-alcoholic Bach flower remedies are also available, so be sure to tell your Bach practitioner that you want non-alcoholic Bach flower remedies.

It is possible to combine a maximum of seven remedies, depending on the type of person and the needs they wish to address. If a crisis mix remedy is added to your personal bottle, it counts as one flower remedy, not five individual ones.

How should I take Bach flower remedies?

You take four drops from your personal bottle, four times a day. The drops are put directly into the mouth.

Bach's crisis mix remedy is taken in the following manner: four drops at a time until the condition improves.

If you want to take any individual flower remedy instead of preparing a personal mix, you should take two drops from the stock bottle, and repeat as needed.

Are there any other ready-made combinations of Bach flower remedies except the one for crisis situations?

The only ready-made combination of Bach flower remedies recommended by The Bach Centre is the one for crisis situations, which contains five flower remedies that help in crisis situations. This combination was put together by Dr. Bach so he could help people in situations when they are experiencing crisis, shock or panic. Its purpose is to provide 'emotional first aid', so that after the crisis, an individual's reaction can be noticed immediately instead of waiting to combine crisis remedies into one therapy.

Many manufacturers produce combinations of remedies for certain problems, such as insomnia, depression, menopausal problems, etc. The advice of The Bach Centre and my advice is not to use such ready-made combinations because it is wrong to make one universal combination for each problem that will be applicable to everyone. It is not the same to make a combination for a person who cannot sleep because they are taking an exam the next morning and for a person who suffers from chronic insomnia. People are not equal when it comes to emotions nor do they react in the same way. To help everyone individually, we need to find the right combination for that person. The Bach practitioner is of great importance because they will help you choose a combination of Bach flower remedies that is specific to you and your ailments.

Pre-prepared combinations that can be bought at the pharmacy and contain several different flower remedies in principle can work, but sometimes the client will see no change. The reason for this is that it sometimes happens that two or three types of remedies from that combination work, while the other remedies in that bottle are superfluous for that person. At the same time, the combination does not contain the other three or four flower remedies a person might need. Therefore, it is more effective to prepare a personal bottle of Bach flower remedies with the help of a Bach practitioner, containing up to seven flower remedies that will be beneficial to that person.

Some Bach flower practitioners use a questionnaire that the client fills out to determine which remedies they would need, or use a pendulum, a muscle test, even randomly drawing cards with pictures of flower remedies, or randomly pulling bottles of flower remedies out of a box. Can any of these methods be used to select flower remedies?

Bach flower practitioners registered at The Bach Centre in England select flower remedies solely on the basis of an interview with a client, which is the way Dr. Bach himself worked. The Bach Centre Code of Ethics strictly prohibits registered Bach flower practitioners from using any method of selecting flower remedies other than selection based on a conversation with a client. You can find a list of registered Bach practitioners on the Bach Centre website[36] to avoid unprofessional selection of flower remedies by non-Bach flower practitioners. Another reason for disapproving of such approaches in counselling is that the person who comes for a consultation becomes 'dependent' on the counsellor to be able to choose the flower remedies for their problems, and the point of Bach's system is for clients to learn to recognise their states and emotions as soon as possible so they themselves can choose and mix flower remedies without the help of an advisor. Using a pendulum, muscle test or other selection technique makes a person dependent on a counsellor.

Of course everyone is free to choose an advisor for Bach flower remedies who suits them, but it is important to know that counsellors who use such non-interview-based selection methods are not registered practitioners at The Bach Centre.

Can Bach flower remedies be taken in coffee, tea or water?

Bach flower remedies can be put in coffee, tea, water and juices, and even in food – and this is how they differ from homeopathic remedies and Schuessler salts. Putting flower remedies in a hot beverage encourages the evaporation of alcohol. This method is recommended for people who do not like or do not want to feel alcohol.

---

[36] https://www.bachcentre.com/en/contact/practitioners/

Can remedies work faster if we do not dilute them with water, but consume them direct from the original bottle?

If you do not dilute them, the alcohol in the remedies will have a stronger taste, and this may give the impression that the remedies are 'stronger', but this is not true. There is no difference in strength and effect between taking flower remedies from your personal bottle and taking flower remedies from the original bottle. But certainly, whoever wants to can take the flower remedies direct from the original bottle.

Can pregnant and breastfeeding women take Bach flower remedies?

Pregnant women can take Bach flower remedies without any problem. The percentage of alcohol present in the remedies is negligible. However, if you are worried about alcohol, it is possible to obtain and make Bach flower remedies without alcohol, or to put the flower remedies into a bottle of water, instead of popping them directly into your mouth from your personal bottle.

Can children and babies take Bach flower remedies?

Children and babies can take Bach flower remedies without a problem. The percentage of alcohol present in the remedies is negligible. But if you are worried about alcohol, it is possible to obtain and make Bach flower remedies without alcohol. The dosage for children and babies is the same as for adults – that is, four drops are taken four times a day. For babies who are breastfeeding, it is best that their mother takes the remedies herself, and the baby will get the remedies through her breast milk. For young children, remedies should always be diluted, using cooled boiled water.

Can Bach flower remedies be taken with medication?

There is usually no problem when taking Bach flower remedies with other medications. The active ingredient in flower remedies is energy from plants, not a physical substance, so it has no influence or effect on other drugs, and does not interfere with them. Neither do drugs interfere with the action of Bach flower remedies. The only thing you should pay attention to is the alcohol used to preserve the remedies. The amount of alcohol in the dose is negligible, but it is still recommended to consult your doctor or pharmacist about taking Bach alcohol-based remedies, especially if you have been advised to avoid alcohol.

Can Bach flower remedies be taken along with Ayurvedic preparations, Schuessler salts and homeopathy?

Simultaneous application is possible. Indeed, homeopaths and Schuessler salt consultants often recommend Bach flower remedies to their clients.

Can Australian Bush flower essences or some other essences be taken at the same time, in addition to Bach flower remedies?

Australian Bush flower essences or some other flower essences *are not a supplement or extension of the Bach flower remedies system*, and are a special and separate method, just like other methods, such as homeopathy or Schuessler salts. Therefore, these or any other essences can be taken freely with Bach flower remedies, if you wish to take them at the same time.

Bach flower remedies form a system of 38 flower remedies set up by the English physician and homeopath, Dr. Edward Bach. They help with 38 different mental states and emotions, and as such form a complete system. Other systems of flower essences, such as Bush flower essences, are not a complement to the set of Bach flower remedies and are considered separate and distinct methods of natural healing. The reason for this is that Dr. Bach was primarily interested in human behaviour and psychology, as well as the mental causes of disease. So he chose plants to treat mental and emotional states and types of people, and did not search for all available medicinal plants in nature. His system covers all human states and emotions, and therefore the system does not need to be expanded.

If you want to use some other essences, you can do so and they will not reduce the effect of Bach flower remedies. However, it is important to keep in mind that these flower essences do not replace or supplement Bach flower remedies.

Is there a possibility of developing an addiction or getting used to Bach flower remedies?

Addiction or dependence is not possible. As long as you feel the need to take the flower remedies, it means that your condition or emotions are not yet balanced out. When you happen to forget to take the flower remedies, or you no longer feel the need to take them, it is just your body telling you that your condition and emotions are now balanced or that some other combination is needed instead of the existing one. The application of Bach flower remedies usually lasts two to three weeks, which is how long your personal bottle often lasts. But sometimes it is necessary to take Bach flower remedies for a longer period, for example three to six months or longer, but even then you will not develop an addiction. If you are afraid that you may become addicted to them, you can stop taking them at any time, and you will see that no side effects will occur as a result. It is not necessary to gradually reduce the doses you take in order to discontinue their use, as is the case with some allopathic medicines. You can completely stop using them at any time, without fear that it will cause unwanted consequences for your body.

How many Bach flower remedies can I take at once?

Usually up to seven flower remedies are taken at the same time. This is the maximum number of remedies that is recommended. It is perfectly normal for people to need more than seven remedies. Some feel they need all the remedies. But it is important that you choose flower remedies only for those emotions and problems that you currently want to solve. We don't use flower remedies for those emotions we felt yesterday, a month ago or a few years ago.

However, although the combination of seven remedies is the recommendation of experts, using eight or nine remedies will not harm you, but will only slow down the action of the remedies if some of those you are taking aren't needed. Bach practitioners are trained to recognise the main flower remedies you need on that particular day and will certainly be able to pick no more than seven remedies, even when you may feel like you need a lot more.

Although Dr. Bach considered the possibility of taking all 38 flower remedies at once in one bottle, he tested the idea and realised that it didn't work. Thus he learned from his experience that most often only six or seven current states or emotions are present in one person. He gave a patient a personal bottle with nine flower remedies in only two cases during his many years of practice.

If I take a remedy for too long, can I develop negative states from that same remedy?

This is not possible. The remedies are completely positive and can in no way cause negative states in a person. There is no risk of so-called proving of a remedy that is specific to homeopathy if the same remedy is taken for too long or too often. Bach flower remedies always have only a positive effect.

How long does it take for the flower remedies to take effect?

The remedy for crisis situations acts quite quickly when used for acute or emergency situations. However, for deep-rooted problems, it may take weeks or months to fully resolve them. It depends more on the person and the problem rather than the speed of action of the flower remedies. Other remedies can also work quickly, but if it is something that bothers you for a long time, the action of the remedies can begin in a few days or weeks, when you will feel the changes. In other words, the flower remedies should act quickly to make you feel better, or even completely relieved of the negative state that is bothering you. But progress is individual.

Dr. Bach stated just that in his lecture on flower remedies: 'Sometimes it takes less time to cure a so-called terrible disease in some people than it takes for some milder diseases in others. It depends more on the person than on the disease itself.'

When should I stop taking Bach flower remedies?

You can stop using Bach flower remedies as soon as the problem that made you start taking them disappears. There is no need to continue taking the remedies unless the problem reoccurs. Also, there is no need for gradual withdrawal from Bach flower remedies, as is required with some other medications. And there is no need to take a certain dose at specific time intervals, as is necessary when administering, for example, antibiotics.

If the condition worsens while taking Bach flower remedies, should I stop using them?

Bach flower remedies do not cause any side effects or worsening of a condition, but it is possible that the remedies stimulate repressed emotions that should be 'purified' before complete healing. If you experience this, talk to your Bach practitioner about replacing the remedies or taking new remedies. Since the remedies have only positive effects, it is not necessary to stop taking them. Also, in cases when you take the wrong remedies you cannot feel any negative effects because the wrong remedies in that case do nothing to the body, nor do they worsen the condition.

Are there combinations of remedies that should never be used?

No. Even remedies that can be characterised as opposites, like Vine and Centaury, sometimes need to be taken simultaneously by the same person. It all depends on the personality and current emotional state of the person.

What if I use my personal combination of Bach flower remedies, and some stressful event happens to me and I need to take some flower remedies that are not in my combination?

If you are currently using your personal combination, which contains fewer than seven flower remedies, you can add the flower remedies you need to your personal bottle. If there are already seven types of flower remedy in your combination, and the flower remedies you need are not in your combination, then feel free to take those flower remedies separately, once or several times that day, until the emotion you feel subsides. When the emotion you felt has subsided, you can continue using the flower remedies from your personal bottle. But if you need more than one type of remedy and your emotional state has changed, then you need to prepare a new personal bottle that matches your current condition, and you should no longer use the old bottle.

Why take four drops of the crisis mix remedy, and two drops of other remedies?

The crisis mix contains a smaller amount of the individual mother tincture of each remedy than an original individual bottle. Therefore, it is necessary to take twice the dose recommended for a single flower remedy.

Do I have to add alcohol to my personal bottle of Bach flower remedies?

Alcohol is used as a preservative because it helps preserve the remedies and prevent evaporation. It is recommended to add alcohol to Bach flower remedies if you do not keep your bottle in a cool place. If you carry it in a bag or pocket, about 5 ml of brandy is quite enough to keep your remedies fresh. If you want to prepare a bottle of flower remedies without alcohol, then keep the bottle in the refrigerator or add one teaspoon of vinegar or glycerine. Bach alcohol-free remedies are also available worldwide for the preparation of your personal combination.

Can devices and radiation negatively affect Bach flower remedies?

No, Bach flower remedies are not as sensitive as homeopathic remedies. They are not affected by airport X-rays, barcode readers, or radiation from cell phones, televisions or computer screens. You can hold them next to your cell phone and go through security X-rays without fear. You can also keep them in the refrigerator. Only avoid heat and direct sunlight due to which the alcohol in the flower remedies can go stale and taste unpleasant.

APPLICATION OF BACH FLOWER REMEDIES DURING EPIDEMICS

As I am finishing this book during the Covid-19 pandemic, here I will single out a few of Dr. Bach's texts that I consider relevant to the state of the world today, and offer some comments and recommendations of my own.

ABOUT FEAR: WHY CAN FEAR WORSEN OR MAKE US MORE SUSCEPTIBLE TO DISEASE?

'In this age the fear of disease has developed until it has become a great power for harm, because it opens the door to those things we dread and makes it easier for their admission. Such fear is really self-interest, for when we are earnestly absorbed in the welfare of others there is no time to be apprehensive of personal maladies. Fear at the present time is playing a great part in intensifying disease, and modern science has increased the reign of terror by spreading abroad to the general public its discoveries, which as yet are but half-truths. The knowledge of bacteria and the various germs associated with disease has played havoc in the minds of tens of thousands of people, and by the dread aroused in them has in itself rendered them more susceptible of attack. While lower forms of life, such as bacteria, may play a part in or be associated with physical disease, they constitute by no means the whole truth of the problem, as can be demonstrated scientifically or by everyday occurrences.'

Edward Bach, *Heal Thyself*, 1931

See how important it is to stay positive! Although the media has warned us to stay home, it is not good to dedicate all our time to watching the news and reading the news about coronavirus on web portals.

WHY DO SOME PEOPLE GET SICK DURING AN EPIDEMIC AND SOME DON'T?

Dr. Bach also gave an answer to the question of why, during epidemics, there are always those who do not succumb to the disease. What is so different about them that prevents them from getting sick? Dr. Bach explains that the answer lies in positive thinking and the power of the mind.

'There is a factor which science is unable to explain on physical grounds, and that is why some people become affected by disease whilst others escape, although both classes may be open to the same possibility of infection. Materialism forgets that there is a factor above the physical plane which in the ordinary course of life protects or renders susceptible any particular individual with regard to disease, of whatever nature it may be. Fear, by its depressing effect on our mentality, thus causing disharmony in our physical and magnetic bodies, paves the way for invasion, and if bacteria and such physical means were the sure and only cause of disease, then indeed there might be but little encouragement not to be afraid. But when we realise that in the worst epidemics only a proportion of those exposed to infection are attacked and that, as we have already seen, the real cause of disease lies in our own personality and is within our control, then have we reason to go about without dread and fearless, knowing that the remedy lies with ourselves. We can put all fear of physical means alone as a cause of disease out of our minds, knowing that such anxiety merely renders as susceptible, and that if we are endeavouring to bring harmony into our personality we need anticipate illness no more than we dread being struck by lightning or hit by a fragment of a falling meteor.'

Edward Bach, Heal Thyself, 1931

In his work *Free Thyself*, from 1932, Dr. Bach again tackled the topic of epidemics:

'We have so long blamed the germ, the weather, the food we eat as the causes of disease; but many of us are immune in an influenza epidemic; many love the exhilaration of a cold wind, and many can eat cheese and drink black coffee late at night with no ill effects. Nothing in nature can hurt us when we are happy and in harmony, on the contrary all nature is there for our use and our enjoyment. It is only when we allow doubt and depression, indecision or fear to creep in that we are sensitive to outside influences.

It is, therefore, the real cause behind the disease, which is of the utmost importance; the mental state of the patient himself, not the condition of his body.'

Edward Bach, Free Thyself, 1932

In the same work, he adds the degrees of healing that are necessary for a person to overcome the disease, if he does become ill.

'There are seven beautiful stages in the healing of disease, these are:

PEACE

HOPE

JOY

FAITH

CERTAINTY

WISDOM

LOVE'

TODAY'S HOSPITAL IN THE AGE OF CORONAVIRUS

The aforementioned stages of healing the disease, however, are not always available to patients in our hospitals.

Bach's works, written between 1931 and 1936, were advanced and ahead of their time. I would personally contend that, today, a lot of his texts remain ahead of their time, even though they were written a little under a century ago. He wrote using simple language, and his works were visionary. He saw the future of healing very differently from how it was practised in his time and how it is practised today.

Throughout the pandemic, via both conventional and social media, we have had the opportunity to read numerous descriptions and see numerous videos of hospitals, where staff in protective equipment are caring for patients isolated in coronavirus wards. Illness, frightening diagnoses, dread and, moreover, loneliness prevail. The patients' loved ones could not reach them – but the pandemic requires sacrifices and necessitates protection of the healthy population. For this reason, family members – both healthy and sick – are going through emotional crises wrought by separation from their loved ones, and fear and concern for the health and lives of those who are sick. The frightening scenes occurring in hospitals, where people die, medical staff are in protective gear and patients on respirators, serve to contribute to an additional fear in patients, which is unfavourable for their mental stability, and yet what is happening in hospitals is the only available solution for their recovery and well-being.

This means that a great deal depends on each individual, who needs to do everything possible to protect both their own health and that of their family, and to maintain the mental health and resilience of the organism with a balanced lifestyle and additional remedies.

Below I describe how Dr. Bach foresaw the conditions in which people would be treated in hospital.

VISION OF DR. EDWARD BACH: THE HOSPITAL OF THE FUTURE

In contrast to what is happening in today's hospitals during this epidemic, we have Dr. Bach's vision of the 'hospital of the future'.

Below I bring you the text of Dr. Bach from the work *Ye Suffer from Yourselves*, which he wrote in 1931:

'Let's look at the hospital of the future for a moment.

It will be a haven of peace, hope and joy. No rush, no noise, completely devoid of all the frightening devices and devices of today, without the unpleasant smells of antiseptics and anaesthetics, and devoid of anything reminiscent of disease and suffering. There will be no frequent temperature measurements and disturbance of the patient's peace; there will be no frequent examinations with stethoscopes and devices that imprint into patients' minds the type of their disease. There will be no continuous heart rate measurement suggesting that the heart is beating fast. All these things prevent the existence of an atmosphere of peace and quiet, which is so necessary for the patient's quick recovery. There will no longer be a need for laboratories because microscopic examinations will no longer be important when we fully realise that we are treating a person, not a disease.

The purpose of all institutions will be to create an atmosphere of peace, hope, happiness and trust. Everything will be done for the purpose of encouraging the patient to forget his illness: to strive for health and at the same time to correct deficiencies in his nature and to understand the lesson to be learned.

Everything in the hospital of the future will be stimulating and beautiful, so that the patient will seek refuge there, and not just a cure for the disease, he will develop a desire to live his life in accordance with the dictates of his Soul.

The hospital will be the mother of the sick, will take him in their arms, comfort and nurture him, give him hope, faith and courage to overcome all difficulties.

The doctor of the future will realise that he is not the one who has the power to heal. But if he devotes his life to the service of his neighbour, studies the human psyche and understands at least part of its essence, if he wants to remove suffering with all his heart and surrender to the healing of the sick, then he will be given the knowledge to guide him and the healing power to remove their pain. Even then, his ability to help others will be proportional to the intensity of his desire and willingness to serve.'

Unfortunately, such a hospital does not yet exist. And I am not sure it ever will.

One day, this will be just an episode from our lives, which we will retell. Because we will weather this and persevere.

SOME REMEDIES I RECOMMENDED

Here I will also tell you about some flower remedies I recommended to be considered by people who had a hard time withstanding self-isolation and the fear of being infected with the virus. In those days, I received frequent enquiries from clients about how to deal with isolation, how to overcome the depression that was taking hold of them, and how to stay positive when bombarded with bad news.

No one had it easy. Our world turned upside down in just a month. No one could tell us how long the situation was going to last and this amplified people's frustrations.

My first recommendation was to consider Walnut. It operates on several different levels. First, it helps people adapt more easily to isolation and to all the rules that we need to adhere to, the so-called 'new normal'. In addition, this flower remedy helps us deal with bad energy and people that are affecting us.

Bach's remedy White Chestnut also helps, if you have problems with unwanted negative thoughts that swirl in the mind, which create negative future scenarios. This remedy will be particularly useful to you if these negative disturbing thoughts are spinning in your head before going to bed. With this remedy you will sleep more peacefully.

If you still sink into a negative mood, Gentian will quickly lift you up from that state, because it gives hope that everything will be fine in the end and that tomorrow will be better than today or yesterday. You will take Gorse if you are immersed in negative thoughts, when you see everything painted in black and when it seems there is no hope of getting out of this situation. Gorse will make you revert to positive thinking and will give you back hope.

During lockdown, many missed socialising the most: hanging out with friends, going out, and even going to school or work. Accordingly, you may need to take Honeysuckle if you tend to reflect on past times in which you could walk freely and enjoy yourself. On the other hand, if you are fantasising about the times when it will be possible for you to go out again, and for moments when people are in the future in their mind, Clematis can help. These two remedies help us stay in the present moment and dedicate ourselves to us, our family and the work tasks (or household chores) before us.

Impatiens is also one of the remedies you might consider in the period of self-isolation. It is suitable for those who have a problem staying in one place, who are impatient, who find it hard to bear the 'captivity' in the house, and those who are counting the days until the end of isolation. Impatiens will be helpful if you fit that description, and should be taken in such situations.

As coronavirus spread, so did fear and panic. In such cases, Bach flower remedies have the power to turn negative emotions into positive.

Here are some of the possible Bach flower remedies that you can consider, to help you cope more easily with isolation, fear and panic:

- Aspen – unknown fear
- Mimulus – fear of disease, fear of death, fear of coronavirus
- Rock Rose – panic fear of the disease
- Red Chestnut – fear and concern for our loved ones, for our children, our parents
- Crab Apple – for the impression that the virus is all around us, for disgust, constantly thinking about possible infection
- Walnut – for protection against external negative influences that affect us

The remedies of your choice should be taken as a personal mix, four drops four times a day, or more often if needed.

APPLICATION OF BACH FLOWER REMEDIES AFTER AN EARTHQUAKE

On 22 March 2020, Croatia's capital city, Zagreb, and its surroundings were hit by a strong earthquake at the peak of the Covid-19 pandemic. As a consequence, in addition to the existing fear and stress due to coronavirus, we also acquired a new fear – the fear of earthquakes. At the time, I posted this text on my blog, to help people recover more easily from this shock. I am conveying the text here too, because it may be useful for future generations or people from other countries after an earthquake.

After the earthquake, many difficult questions arose in people's minds: are we safe in our own homes while we sleep, rest, perform daily activities? Can we now peacefully leave our children alone in the house and go to work, knowing we are not safe from an earthquake?

Immediately after the earthquake, citizens ran to the meadows, parked their cars on the meadows, sat in their cars or just stood in the open air, fearing that a new wave of earthquakes would start at any moment.

Some packed their things and left town. Huge lines formed in front of the gas stations. People started fleeing the city.

Messages arrived early in the morning, everyone calling their loved ones to check on them.

So here is list of possible Bach flower remedies that can help in these moments of stress, fear and panic:

- Star of Bethlehem – for shock
- Rock Rose – for panic
- Mimulus – for fear of earthquakes
- Red Chestnut – for fear and concern for our loved ones
- Gentian – for discouragement after an unpleasant event
- Cherry Plum – to stay calm despite great stress
- Crisis mix, which contains five pre-selected stress remedies

There are only a few possible remedies, as each person is an individual and everyone can react differently, so keep this in mind when choosing your own remedies.

Since that earthquake I have heard that many sleep on the living room couch, dressed in tracksuits and sneakers. Some do not sleep all night out of fear, and wait for the morning to peacefully close their eyes and get some rest. I also read about a child who wants to sit in the car all the time and is afraid to be in the house. There are many too who hear the sound of the earthquake in their head or constantly relive in their mind the moments when the earthquake happened. Some people were reminded of the war that took place in this area in the early 1990s, and it stirred up old shocks and fears. Some were alone at home and now fear even more – both earthquakes and loneliness. Above all, some were killed in the quake, and some had their homes significantly damaged or destroyed. All of these people experienced a great shock.

Be sure to consider all the specifics of your situation and all the emotions you are currently feeling while choosing remedies for your personal bottle.

DR. BACH'S INSTRUCTIONS FOR THOSE WHO WISH TO HELP OTHERS AND BECOME HEALERS

'Healing with the clean, pure, beautiful agents of Nature is surely the one method of all which appeals to most of us, and deep down in our inner self, surely there is something about it that rings true indeed: something which tells us – this is Nature's way and is right.'

* * *

'The whole principle of Healing by this method is so simple as can be understood by almost everyone, and even the very Herbs themselves can be gathered and prepared by any who take delight in such.'

* * *

'There are amongst us in almost every town or village some who have to a lesser or greater degree the desire to be able to help in illness; to be able to relieve the suffering and heal the sick, but from circumstances have been prevented from becoming doctors or nurses, and have not felt that they were able to carry out their desire or mission.

These herbs place in their hands the power to heal amongst their own families, friends and all around them.

In addition to their occupation, they are enabled in their spare time to do a very great amount of good, as many are so doing today; and there are some who have even given up their work to devote all their time to this form of healing.

It means to those who always had an ideal, a dream of relieving the suffering, that it has been made possible for them, whether it be but their own household or on a wider scale.'

***

'It is not the disease that is of importance. It is the patient; the way in which he or she is affected which is our true guide to healing.'

***

'Again to impress upon you that there is no need of scientific knowledge necessary when treating with these herbs: not even the name of the illness or disease is required. It is not the disease that matters: it is the patient. It is not what the patient has. It is not the disease, so-called, that really is the important thing to treat; because the same disease may cause different results in different people. If the effects were always the same in all people, it would be easy to know what the name of the disease was: but this is not so; and this is the reason why often in medical science it is so difficult to give a name to the particular complaint from which a patient is suffering.'

***

'Once again, let it be made quite certain that, whether it is being run down, or not quite oneself; Whether trying to prevent a disease; whether it is a short illness or a long, the principle is the same – treat the patient; treat the patient according to the mood, according to the character, the individuality, and you cannot go wrong.'

* * *

'Now, it is just the same principle of treatment in long illness as when it is slight and short or only even threatened.'

* * *

'... it is the work of spiritual healers and physicians to give, in addition to material remedies, the knowledge to the suffering of the error of their lives, and of the manner in which these errors can be eradicated, and so to lead the sick back to health and joy.'

* * *

'Suffice it to say that there is one [remedy, author's note] for every mood which can be an opposition to our happy joyful selves. And all that is necessary is to know that mood or moods present in the patient and give the Remedy or Remedies which remove them.'

* * *

'This work of healing has been done, and published and given freely so that people like yourselves can help yourselves, either in illness or to keep well and strong. It requires no science; only a little knowledge and sympathy and understanding of human nature, which is usual with almost all of us.'

* * *

'Think once again the joy this brings, to any one who wants to be able to do something for those who are ill, to be able to help even those where medical science can do no more; it gives to them the power to be healers amongst their fellows.'

* * *

'And, once again, the important point is this: that wonderful as it may seem, relieve your patient of the mood or moods such as are given in this system of healing, and your patient is better.'

* * *

BACH FLOWER REMEDIES FOR ANIMALS

Just as humans can benefit greatly from the application of Bach flower remedies, they can also be used for animals. The only difference is the dosage and the fact that the animal cannot say what is bothering it, so the owner must talk about it. The owner and Bach's practitioner will observe the animal, and based on observations and experience in the application of the flower remedies, a combination of flower remedies suitable for the animal will be prepared.

To choose flower remedies for an animal, we need to consider:

- temperament (propensity towards certain behaviours and usual level of activity)
- behaviour (reaction to external factors)
- personality of an animal
- specific behaviour of a certain animal species

Dosages for animals

There are two methods for determining dosage for small animals (dogs, cats, rabbits, etc.):

1. the flower remedies can be placed directly in the water the animal drinks, or on a suitable pet treat

2. a bottle of personal mix can be prepared, so flower remedies are added from that bottle to the food or water that the animal takes

For small animals the rules are the same as for humans. Add four drops of crisis mix remedy and two drops of other remedies in the personal mix. This is taken four times a day, four drops, the same as for humans.

Dosage methods for large animals (horses, cows, elephants, etc.):

1. ten drops are added to a bucket of water, or

2. four drops are put on an animal treat

This is taken four times a day or as often as needed.

Examples – how to determine the remedies needed

Why is the dog barking?

- it is afraid (Mimulus, Rock Rose)

- possessively protects its owner (Chicory)

- protects its territory and shows its dominance (Vine)

- another animal attacks it and it feels threatened (Centaury)

Examples of behaviour when an animal is sick:

- seeks the attention of the owner (Chicory)

- has a sad look (Willow)

- wants to be the centre of attention of all household members (Heather)

There are two remedies that you will surely give to your animals often – Walnut and Star of Bethlehem.

Significance of Walnut remedy application for animals

This flower remedy provides durability and protection from external influences.

The most important flower remedy when a pet comes to your home for the first time!

These are flower remedies for easier adjustment in periods of change/transition, if there is difficulty adapting to a new situation:

- a new family member, the birth of a child
- moving to a new apartment or city
- going on a trip with the owners
- staying in the house with another person while the owners go on a trip

Walnut is a remedy for protection against external influences, for example:

- the household members are nervous, angry or sick
- a visit from a person who does not like the animal

Significance of the application of Star of Bethlehem remedy for animals

- shock after bad news, loss of a loved one, horror after an accident and the like
- shock due to a new environment

- shock due to moving to a new city or apartment
- shock after a day at a dog hotel or other caregiver's place
- something ugly happened during walking, another animal bit them
- shock when going to the vet
- sudden sound or shock when an animal reacts to this as a shock
- shock due to death or change of the owner

Our two English Bulldogs, Rocky and Rambo, love Bach flower remedies, homeopathy and tissue salts.

BACH FLOWER REMEDIES FOR PLANTS

For plants, you will certainly often use the crisis mix, but it is equally important to give selected individual flower remedies in certain situations.

How do you choose flower remedies when plants cannot tell you about their feelings? Simply use your intuition and imagination when choosing flower remedies. Observe the plant and the circumstances in which it is located to help you figure out its condition.

Examples

- use Walnut when the plant is exposed to changes – for example, due to temperature changes, transfer from one room to another, during transplatation, re-potting, etc. – if you see problems in adaptation to new environment

- Star of Bethlehem should be used when the plant is exposed to shocks – for example, adverse weather conditions

- Crab Apple may be useful when a plant is attacked by parasites, as we may assume it is feeling dirty

Dosage for plants

Add ten drops to the watering can if you water all the plants with the same flower remedies.

For an individual plant – put two drops of a single remedy and/or four drops of crisis mix in the water with which you water the plant, or spray the plant with water to which you have added some chosen flower remedies or crisis mix. If the plant must not be over-watered, we can put a little water with the drops on a small teaspoon, and water the plant with only that one teaspoon.

HOW TO RECOGNISE INDIVIDUAL BACH FLOWER REMEDIES ON SOCIAL NETWORKS

Since people today, and especially young people, mostly spend a lot of time on social networks, I decided to analyse states and types of people based on their posts and behaviour in the virtual world, and connected Bach flower remedies with them on this basis.

Bach flower remedies and their application	Indication for application
Agrimony – hiding worries and problems behind a happy face	Does not like to publish anything private about themselves, so they just post funny stories and pictures. If they do publish pictures of themselves, they are all smiling and happy pictures – announcements of an ideal life.
Aspen – unknown fear	Posting texts on unknown fears.
Beech – intolerance	Criticise others in comments, and don't mince their words.

Centaury – inability to say no	Likes posts out of decency, things they wouldn't actually like. Accept friend requests they do not really want, again out of politeness, not to turn them down.
Cerato – lack of confidence in their own decisions	When making a decision, they ask for advice via social media.
Cherry Plum – fear of losing control and reason	Posts and comments in which they declare their desire or intention to do something uncontrollably.
Chestnut Bud – constant repetition of the same mistakes	Repeating the same mistakes while posting content.
Chicory – selfish and possessive love	Include their partner in all posts: 'XY is with YY at ZZ location ...'
Clematis – excessive daydreaming about the future	When on social media they forget about the present and the time. They follow pages about travel, cruises or other things they dream about.
Crab Apple – for cleaning, self-loathing	Crab Apple people don't like to post pictures of themselves and don't allow others to tag them. Their profile picture does not show them.
Elm – overburdened with responsibilities	Elm complains that it is overburdened with responsibilities.
Gentian – discouragement after failure	After the post did not achieve the desired response or popularity, they are discouraged and fear how their future posts will be viewed.
Gorse – loss of hope, despair	They deactivate their profile when faced with a situation that is unfavourable to them.
Heather – excessive focus on oneself	Publishes pictures of everything – what they ate, where they were, who they were with and, if they have children, then they publish pictures of the children in all clothing combinations and all situations.
Holly – hatred, envy and jealousy	Haters. They write comments full of hatred and envy. They browse through other people's profiles with jealousy.

Honeysuckle – excessive thinking about the past	They publish past memories.
Hornbeam – tired of the thought of a job	Spends time on social networks, while postponing job responsibilities.
Impatiens – impatience	Does not read posts that are too long.
Larch – lack of self-confidence	Seeks the confirmation of others for something they have done, and about which they are unsure themselves.
Mimulus – everyday fears, of familiar things	Post about their fears that can be named.
Mustard – depression that occurs for no reason	Gloomy posts even though it is a beautiful day and even though nothing negative is happening in their life. Positive and depressing posts alternate.
Oak – excessive work beyond the limits of endurance	Oak may not have a social network account if he sees them as a waste of time, or he is running local support groups.
Olive – fatigue after mental or physical exertion	Olive does not have the strength at the end of the day yet to open and browse through social media because they are too tired.
Pine – guilt	Feels guilty about the posts or messages they write over social media.
Red Chestnut – excessive concern for the welfare of loved ones	Publishes warning posts about forthcoming dangers.
Rock Rose – panic and terror	Spreads panic on social networks – for example, a comet is approaching that will hit the Earth, poisonous toys for children are on sale, etc.
Rock Water – self-imposed restrictions, rigid attitudes, self-punishment	Publishes pictures and posts of themselves and their activities, hoping that others will follow their positive example.
Scleranthus – inability to make a decision	Cannot decide which picture to publish.
Star of Bethlehem – shock	Posts about something that shook them.

Sweet Chestnut – a pronounced mental agony, there seems to be no way out	They publish painful stories and comments that show agony.
Vervain – excessive enthusiasm	Social media activist. Advocates for a certain activity, method, lifestyle, etc.
Vine – domination over others and inflexibility	A parent who controls children's social networks or a partner who controls what their partner posts on social media.
Walnut – protection from the unwanted influence of others, and help to adapt in times of change	Susceptible to trends on social media and publishes posts that are popular, even though they do not feel good to them.
Water Violet – isolation and loneliness	Water Violet neither publishes their photos nor anything about themselves. A person who follows the posts of others but rarely likes someone's posts.
White Chestnut – unwanted thoughts that spin in your head and cause mental torture	Everything they read spins negatively in their head, and causes mental anguish and torture.
Wild Oat – uncertainty when choosing a life direction	Follows a few pages of interest and hopes this will help him/her choose a direction.
Wild Rose – surrender, reconciliation with destiny, apathy	Reluctance and apathy regardless of the positive examples and posts of other people.
Willow – self-pity, resentment, resentment of others	Comments of indignation, publishes sad stories.

RECOMMENDATIONS FOR FURTHER STUDY OF THE WORK OF DR. BACH

For your future study of the teachings of Dr. Bach, it is fundamental to read these written works on Bach flower remedies and on the philosophy of the causes of disease:

- *Heal Thyself*
- *Ye Suffer from Yourselves*
- *Free Thyself*
- *The Twelve Healers and Other Remedies*

The book ***Heal Thyself*** contains a series of wisdoms with which Dr. Bach was familiar at the time. His theses that illness arises as a result of our personality's incompatibility with the dictates of our soul, and as a result of unrooted defects in our personality, prompt us to wonder how we can still progress on our path and what else we can do to help other people and, ultimately, the world.

The text ***Free Thyself*** contains early descriptions of remedies, from the phase when Dr. Bach had not yet discovered all the plants and concluded his research, and is a valuable text for anyone who wants to know more about his work. It is important to note here that in this text it is necessary to carefully read all the prefaces and notes written by the staff of The Bach Centre, which are found in the footnotes throughout the text, because they indicate the differences between the descriptions of individual remedies provided in these early records and the final descriptions given by Dr. Bach when he concluded the system.

The final descriptions of the 38 flower remedies can be found in the work *The Twelve Healers and Other Remedies* and are still today the main guide in the selection of flower essences by practitioners around the world.

The work *Ye Suffer from Yourselves* builds on the philosophy presented in *Heal Thyself.* It is intended primarily for homeopaths, but it is a valuable record of Dr. Bach's vision of what the treatment system should look like, how doctors and homeopaths should work with patients, and how hospitals should be organised and arranged for patients so they could find in them peace, refuge and health.

Dr. Bach has incorporated many personal experiences into his works and, although they are not clearly highlighted in the book, we can recognise them if we read carefully and pay attention. He wanted to share his wisdom with the whole world.

It is important to note that Dr. Bach himself suffered a serious illness when, in 1917, he was given only three more months to live. He lived another 19 years from that day, and he spent all those years working with great zeal, looking for remedies from nature – completely simple and harmless – that would alleviate the suffering of the human race. In his works, Dr. Bach describes the importance of discovering and following one's own unique life path. And he also emphasised this from his own experience because it was the realisation of his life mission that cured him and kept him alive through all those years of his search for medicinal plants. Therefore, his works, advanced for the time when he lived, today give clear guidelines to people around the world on how to maintain health and happiness, and how to find and follow their life path.

Whether you have ever tried Bach flower remedies or not, whether you intend to ever try them, whether you believe in natural healing methods or not, this is a valuable read for each of us! Because Dr. Bach talks here about the life situations we all go through – about our attachments, about the relationship between parents and children, about choosing our profession and recognising our life vocation, about human flaws and virtues, and much more.

Dr. Bach's works should be read slowly and calmly, word for word, so you may recognise in them the words you need today to find a solution or comfort for your problems and troubles. Valuable advice and examples will surely be etched in your memory because Dr. Bach vividly describes each of his theses and supports them with examples from life and the world.

The above texts are available in English in separate editions. The original works in English can be downloaded free of charge from the Bach Centre website at www.bachcentre. com, as can translations into numerous world languages, including the Croatian translation of Dr. Bach's works rendered by Ana Klikovac PhD. The latter can also be downloaded free of charge from the website of the Annah Centre for Homeopathy and Health Support: www.annah.hr.

I wish you a happy and pleasant further study of the system of Bach flower remedies and the work of Dr. Edward Bach!

Ana Klikovac PhD

... relieve your patient of the mood or moods such as are given in this system of healing, and your patient is better.

Dr. Edward Bach, *The Wallingford Lectures*, 1936

ACKNOWLEDGEMENTS

And at the end of this book, I want to express gratitude.

First of all, I am thankful that God's hand wrote this plan for me and that Dr. Bach 'chose' me to spread his wisdom. I wasn't looking for the remedies, at least not consciously. I did not wander the spiritual paths looking for a method that would take me further and higher. The remedies found me! Therefore, with all my soul's might I believe and feel that it is my mission to do this and that Dr. Bach chose me personally precisely because of my Vervain type who gives me the enthusiasm and gift of speech to spread and teach this method.

I am thankful to my husband Saša, who always unreservedly believed in me and supported my every idea, no matter how implausible it sometimes seemed, and who always believed that I would succeed whenever I undertook something new and, from my perspective, big. He was the first to read this book; he reviewed and read everything in detail several times, and his advice and contributions enriched this work so it could be the best version of what I wanted to convey to you. This book would not have existed if my husband had not constantly encouraged and inspired me to write this work that will be of help to many! It is solely to his merit that in this book I share many details of our private lives, without which this book would be merely arid theory and just another in the series of books on Bach flower remedies. His vision was that this book should be an honest and open story about my and our journey with Bach flower remedies. Thus, his contribution and support to every person who will feel better after reading this book are built in to this book! Equally, his support for my intention to do what I do and help others is his concrete contribution to the well-being of the people who turn to me for help.

I am grateful to my children, Helena, Eva and Ante, who inspired me to start using and implementing these methods. I am proud of them because they are independent, distinct, unique, and they love and support one another. I deeply believe and expect that both they and their children will one day have all of these methods available as recognised and effective approaches, alongside classical medicine.

One more thank you, to my daughters Helena and Eva, who made some beautiful drawings of Bach flower remedies for me when I first opened my homeopathic centre, and which I am now using on the cover of this book. By giving me their approval to use these drawings, they have contributed to my vision that this book will be the story of our family's journey with Bach flower remedies. Eva always accompanied me on my trips to The Bach Centre in England, knows every flower from the garden there and was only 12 when she completed the Level 1 course on Bach flower remedies. My entire family was with me at The Bach Centre on the special occasion when I studied to become a licensed teacher. I am happy to say that, today, both Helena and Eva hold their Level 2 certificates in Bach flower remedies, as does my husband. And I am sure that my son Ante will study these remedies in more depth too when he is older, as they are already his daily support in his handball successes.

I also thank all those wonderful souls who have left their profound mark on my life, and without whom I would not be where I am today.

Also, I thank my parents who decided to bring me into this world, who created me and guided me during my childhood the best they could. I thank my mom, who spent a full nine months in bed for me to be born. I thank my dad, who has encouraged me ever since I was little to engage in lifelong learning and diligent work, while at the same time providing me with an unlimited budget for buying books since I have always loved reading. I learned from my father that with diligent and persistent work in life you can achieve the seemingly impossible, and that material and spiritual rewards always come as the result of dedicated work. I learned from my mother how important it is to be supportive of my husband – at all times and in everything – and that this togetherness is the foundation of a long-lasting marriage. I wish to thank them for all the life lessons they have taught me. I believe both my mom and dad today are proud of me, my accomplishments and of my family.

I am happy to have an older sister because this meant that I received an invaluable gift: I became an aunt at the age of 11. I enjoyed babysitting my nieces, ironing their diapers, feeding them and pushing them on a swing. Thanks to the two of them, I learned that the most beautiful – and most important – task in the world is to take care of children. By looking after my two nieces, I learned at a very early age that I could be, and wanted to be, the best mom to my own children. My nieces were my 'practice' and the source of my childhood happiness. Thank you to my sister Silvija for everything I have learned through her children and her story.

I thank my mother-in-law Dragica and my father-in-law Branko for their attention and the support I have received from them, and for their love for their grandchildren.

I thank Štefica, Tomaš and their Ivana, who enriched my life and made it more beautiful.

I thank dear Anita Moorjani, a well-known and inspiring author, a fan of Bach flower remedies, who chose me to be her homeopath precisely because of my story. When we first met and when I told her the story of how I became a homeopath, she was thrilled and told me that I should definitely write a book in which I will describe the turning point in my life, and thus encourage others to follow their path bravely and to embark on a path of *change*! She immediately told me that she wanted me to be her personal homeopath – hers and Danny's, her husband's. I immediately directed her to my website, where she could read more about me and my way of working. She replied: 'I don't need to read anything. I can already see what you are like and I want you to be my homeopath.' It was on that day that the foundations were laid for the materialisation of this book of mine. Personally, I think that the late Dr. Wayne W. Dyer had something to do with all this. It is fascinating that the first book I bought at the bookstore when I embarked on my personal and professional transformation was Dr. Dyer's book, *Change*! Given his importance in the life of Anita Moorjani, and the inspiration I felt a long time ago while reading his book, I am sure that he is very pleased, somewhere up there, that today Anita and I cooperate so nicely and I sincerely thank him for his 'spiritual intervention'! Thank you, dear Anita, for confirming my mission by participating in the making of this book, and for selflessly promoting both my work and the book.

I am grateful to The Bach Centre for the many years of considerate and professional cooperation and I thank all my teachers who guided me through my education there. I had a wonderful mentor at Level 1, Christine Woodham, who was the first to formally teach me about the fundaments of the Bach flower remedies system, and who commented on my assignments with a great deal of attention and warmth. I still hold her mentoring in fond memory, and I hereby thank her for the intensity of her dedication. She opened the door for me to further explorations of Dr. Bach's teachings and I am happy to have had her as a mentor. The majority of the other teachings I studied with Lynn Macwhinnie, whom I affectionately call 'Bach flower remedies supreme teacher'. Lynn is a teacher towards whom you should feel pure awe, given her status at The Bach Centre, her enormous knowledge of Bach flower remedies, and the fact that she learned about the remedies from Nora Weeks herself. Lynn is a teacher who requires that you demonstrate work, effort and knowledge, and she will always have my respect for that.

Many thanks to Judy Ramsell Howard and to all who have maintained this system in practice today and throughout history, and spread it around the world. My gratitude goes to The Bach Centre for insisting on strict guidelines for the work of practitioners and teachers, which ensure consistency in the work and the application of flower remedies in all countries of the world, thus preserving the legacy of Dr.

Bach. I am proud to be a part of all this and to contribute to the spreading of Dr. Bach's teachings.

I would like to thank Stefan Ball, director of The Bach Centre, who made the effort to read this book, thoroughly word for word, and gave me his expert suggestions and comments on the text. He thus fulfilled my wish that the book should be reviewed before publication by an expert from The Bach Centre, to make sure that I had not violated or misinterpreted the teachings of our esteemed Dr. Bach. Before sending this book for printing, I respected absolutely every suggestion I received from Stefan Ball and made all the necessary adaptations, wherever needed, and I believe that a book edited in this way will now more easily reach all those who cry for help and the knowledge it contains. May this book find its way to everyone who needs it, precisely at the moment when they need it, in the same way the information about Bach flower remedies magically reached me!

I would like to thank my Croatian editor, Sandra Pocrnić Mlakar, who recognised the quality and potential of this book, and readily decided to help it see the light of day. Her advice was most helpful in structuring the book.

Many thanks to Dr. Metka Regan who encouraged me when I needed it most, who opened the world of homeopathy to me and recognized the talent of a homeopath in me.

I thank my friend Vesna Dedović, who was Dr. Bach's 'mediator', who recognised Bach flower remedies as the right method for me and carried out her mission to provide me with information about this miraculous method.

I would like to thank my long-term trusted collaborators, Đurđica Margetić and Polonca Kolmačić, who gave their professional contribution, read the book from the point of view of a registered Bach practitioner and prepared reviews of the work.

My colleague from India, Dr. Soni Udasi, is also a special associate of mine, as she is assisting me in my international projects. Her efforts in helping to ensure that this book reaches a wide international audience are much appreciated.

Beautiful India, which my husband and I adore, where I teach homeopathy as part of the faculty at the homeopathic academy 'The Other Song', has also taught me numerous life lessons. Thank you, India, for proudly practising all these methods for decades, and a great many thanks to all its homeopathic doctors who are a stronghold and an example to us in the West.

Here I wish to express my gratitude to Dr. Rajan Sankaran, who opened horizons for me with his theories in homeopathy and showed me the beauty and logic of modern homeopathy. The trust he placed in me by choosing me as his collaborator and teacher of his methods solidified my mission to spread homeopathy and related methods.

Since India holds a special place in my heart, God made it possible for me that this book would be published in the English language by renowned India-based publishing house and specialist in homeopathic literature, B. Jain Publishers. My heartfelt thanks go to its director, Manish Jain, who expressed his sincere desire to publish this book 'written from the heart' and distribute it worldwide.

I thank my clients who have trusted me all these years, and asked for my help in choosing their remedies and homeopathy. I also thank all those who have learned these wonderful and noble methods from me.

I thank too all those clients, friends and family members whose examples I selected in order to enrich this book with practical real-life stories. Let their examples serve as a guiding force and inspiration to others who have yet to achieve a happy and balanced life.

Ana Klikovac
Zagreb, 1 January 2021

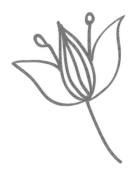

LITERATURE LIST

1. Bach, E., *Free Thyself* (1932)

2. Bach, E., *Heal Thyself* (1931)

3. Bach, E., *Let Us Be Ourselves*, The Bach Centre (2014)

4. Bach, E., *The Story of the Travellers and Other Remedy Stories* (1933, 1934, 1935)

5. Bach, E., *The Twelve Healers and Other Remedies* (1933)

6. Bach, E., *The Wallingford Lectures* (1936)

7. Bach, E., *Two More Essentials*, The Bach Centre (2014)

8. Bach, E., *Ye Suffer from Yourselves* (1931)

9. Ball, S., *Principles of Bach Flower Remedies*, Singing Dragon (2013)

10. Howard, J., *The Bach Flower Remedies Step by Step: A Complete Guide to Selecting and Using the Remedies*, Vermilion (2005)

11. Macwhinnie, L., *Emotional Wisdom with Bach Flower Remedies*, eBookPartnership.com (2014)

12. Moorjani, A., *What if This is Heaven?*, Hay House (2016)

13. Sankaran, R., *Dog, Yogi, Banjan Tree*, Homeopathic Medical Publishers, India (2017)

14. Sankaran, R., *The Sensation in Homeopathy*, 2nd edition, Homoeopathic Medical Publishers (2004)

15. Weeks, N., *The Medical Discoveries of Edward Bach Physician*, The C.W. Daniel Company Limited (1975)

INTERNET SOURCES

- The Bach Centre, www.bachcentre.com.

- University College London Hospitals, www.uclh.nhs.uk, 1 November 2019.

ABOUT THE AUTHOR

Ana Klikovac PhD received her doctoral degree in 2011 at the Faculty of Economics, University of Zagreb, on the topic 'The role of auditing in fraud detection as a prerequisite for the stability of the capital market'. She received her master's degree from the same faculty in 2006 on the topic 'The impact of harmonisation of financial reporting in the European Union on financial reporting in the Republic of Croatia'. From 2006 to 2017 she taught courses in the field of accounting and auditing at a higher education institution and was the head of the graduate study programme Accounting, Auditing and Taxes. She is a certified internal auditor, a specialist in the field of the economy.

She lives and works in Zagreb. She is the owner of the company Annah d.o.o. for homeopathy and health support, where she provides counselling and education in the field of natural healing methods. She is also the owner of the company ASHUH j.d.o.o., whose primary activity is aimed at promoting homeopathy, organising international seminars and other international projects.

She is a certified homeopath. During her education, she visited many world authorities in the field of homeopathy and in her work she uses several different homeopathic approaches. She completed the programme of classical and French homeopathy in Zagreb. At The Other Song International Academy of Advanced Homeopathy, in India, she completed her clinical practice and professional development, and specialised in working according to the Sensation Method and the 8-Box Method of homeopathy.

She completed her education on Bach flower remedies at The Bach Centre in England, where she is a registered practitioner (BFRP). She also completed a teacher programme at The Bach Centre, thus becoming the first certified Level 1 and Level 2 teacher in Croatia.

She has translated a number of works written by Dr. Edward Bach into Croatian, and prepared and edited the book *Heal Thyself and Other Complete Works by Dr. Edward Bach* (*Izliječi sebe i ostali kompletni radovi dr. Edwarda Bacha*, Harša, 2015), which made Dr. Bach's works available in Croatian, united in one book.

She is a consultant and teacher for Schuessler tissue salts and facial analysis. She is a certified practitioner for Australian Bush Flower Essences. She is an accredited practitioner of the Buteyko breathing method.

She is a faculty member and representative of The Other Song International Academy of Advanced Homeopathy of Dr. Rajan Sankaran, in India.

She is married and the mother of three children.

For more information about Ana Klikovac and her work, please visit her websites:

www.anaklikovac.com

www.ashuh.eu

www.annah.hr

NOTES